From Darkness to Light

Walter Gird

Order this book online at www.trafford.com
or email orders@trafford.com

Most Trafford titles are also available at major online book retailers.

Printed in the United States of America.

ISBN: 978-1-4669-5003-0 (sc)
ISBN: 978-1-4669-5005-4 (hc)
ISBN: 978-1-4669-5004-7 (e)

Library of Congress Control Number: 2012914070

Trafford rev. 08/03/2012

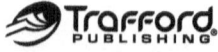 www.trafford.com

North America & international
toll-free: 1 888 232 4444 (USA & Canada)
phone: 250 383 6864 ♦ fax: 812 355 4082

Acknowledgement

And

Thanks

My Daughter Maureen Lillian Henning who was the co-editor of the book. Her unwavering belief in me and its success have been our driving force.

I acknowledge her for that.

Note

All sketches of self are done by the author in pencil.

Prologue

It is an effort to bring a message of hope though a true life story. The life and times of alias "ramasemong" the laughing Hyena, a cancer patient Walter Gird, that's me.

To make this story interesting I have sketched a background of the post 1950's, life as a young boy on the Free State farms during that little known period. As a young lad I had a most stress free existence one could imagine, free as a flying dove above those very hills described.

As an adolescent, I indivertibly landed up in a Roman Catholic Church Seminary. Thinking that I had a higher calling in that direction, it was not to be. After getting married I worked on different types of mines in South Africa. Some incidents in my narrative are what happened to me then. A cause for stress, a prelude to a life threatening disease called cancer. At the age of 59 I was diagnosed with having Lymph Gland Cancer, "Hodgensons" the slow type. As in the past crises, I would look for the positive when the negative was present. It was different now, my life dependent on it, I had to keep a positive mind set all times and try to be aggressive against a life threatening enemy cancer. I believe that if it was not for my positive set of mind and God's strength I would not have survived the chemo therapies sessions and every emotion that is connected with this ordeal.

Contents

Pages

Chapter 1
Mining Stress

Chapter 1   Mining stress

Prologue

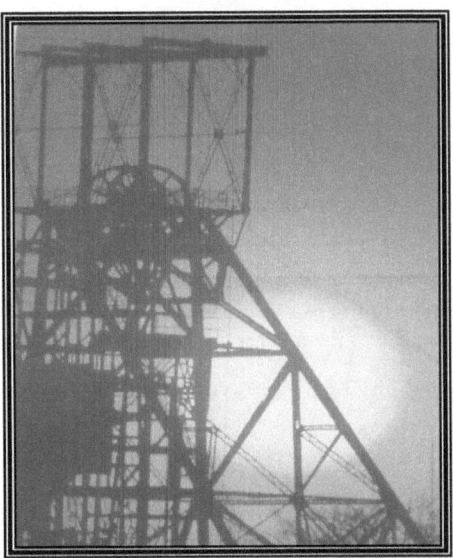

To be a miner deep in the bowels of the earth is a stress factor. The environment is unnatural. The pitch blackness you work in, the excessive heat conditions, heat stroke, falling hanging, the greatest killer, difficult physical conditions for your body to function, poor communication between workers and management, blacks far firm homelands, living in over crowded compounds or hostels. Alcoholism, prostitutes, continual fear of injury all made life difficult. This was the environment I worked in for 35 years. I worked on most of the major mines, coal, diamond, platinum, and gold mining from the deepest on the Rand to the Goldfields of Welkom.

I started my mining career as a learner miner, learning all the physical work to be done by black miner-workers. Lashing stuff by hand, tipping the gold the bear reef, by means of pushing half ton coco-pans, through winding passages or gullies with small rails. When the full hopper arrived at the center gully it was tipped by had into it. A moving scraper would pull the stuff to the tip. Other duties were blasting, making areas safe to work in, installing support by means of sticks or packs, I was super fit. In Welkom I studied further and massed the mine overseers' exam, and was promoted to shift boss or foreman. Pressure was the name of the game. The daily call, or blasting, or the tonnage to be tipped would determine whether you would stay or be fired for incompetence or relegated to night shift.

A typical Day: Stress in the dark

As a young shift Boss I remember the following work related incident in a typical underground situation I expected a "visit or inspection" by the Mine Captain that day. When he arrived he shouted "Hyena, come here!" This was a name he gave to me because I had a high pitch giggle when I laughed or got nervous. He was to me a terrifyingly big man, with a long waxed mustache. My dad had a similar one, but the similarity ended there. My dad being short, strong and muscular, handsome, as a matter of fact he came first in the longest wax mustache competition in the Free State years before.

My bosses name was known as Satan with a long A. "Why is the work not completed, Mr. Hyena?" He roared. I answered "the night shift did not complete cleaning". "Bull shit!" he answered. "You will see the manager and pay a fine when you come out, do you understand." Before I could answer he turned to go. Unfortunately standing too close was the team leader, unexpectedly got a back hand. Off they went, the boss with his assistant called a pikanin, out they went, two cap lamps one behind the other until they both disappeared around the bend in the haulage or tunnel.

On surface that afternoon after showering I met the Team leader Thabo, much afraid of the coming charges in the Managers office. I assured him in Sotho that I would win the case, and that he must not worry. He told me that I did not know Satan, much feared by all. At the hearing the Manager heard Satan's story. He asked me what did I plea. "Not guilty" I answered. "Why?" He answered, "Because I did my job, got my call and had no accidents for the day." He was very surprised and asked Satan why my story was different to his, caught unawares, thinking after the night shift set back I had not getting my call. The manager, with drew the charges and congratulated me on work well done, and said I could go. Outside waited Thabo hoping against the worst. On hearing the good news, said he would go and have a beer on "Ramasemong" the father of the fields.

A close shave: Flying rocks

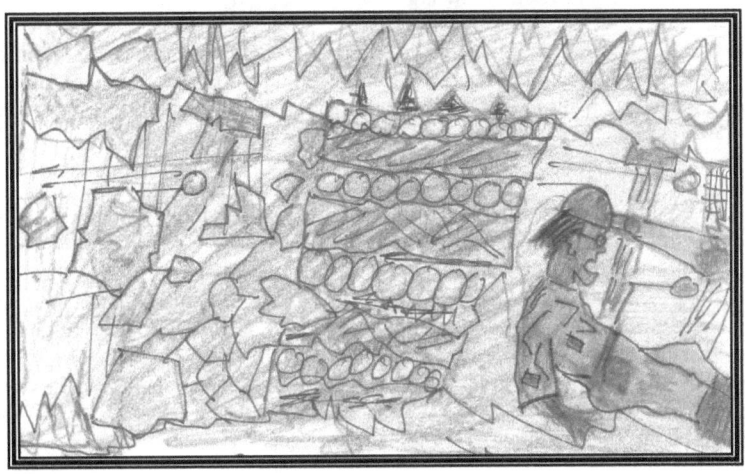

As a young miner I worked on many different mines and was like an adventure to me, different people, and different methods. The deepest and hottest were the gold mines on the Rand. At that time ERPM was the deepest and that's where I worked as a miner. The easiest way to explain the story is first to tell and explain the workings and the environment of how a very deep and hot gold mine function and operate. Because of the depth, the configuration of the faces being must be mined in a certain method. The long wall method was used, meaning to try and mine +_ 300m in a line, each panel divided into 30m panels. Leaving a panel behind would cause geological stress and in turn because a rock fall or worse a seismic event, a great danger to human life should it happen.

I was assigned the bottom panel being the most important leading the rest of the other 9 panels above, lying at a degree of 30 degrees. All the panels were blasted daily so that they could move forward uniformly with out abutments left behind as explained. One pay day every one is in a rush to go out early. The cage would come early. Most of the holes to be charged up were already drilled. The miners assistant myself and the Team leader were busy with this operation and most of the gang had left the station.

Unfortunately the bottom rock drill broke down; the delay would be a mitigating factor to near tragic event that would follow. It was critical time wasted, a great frustration, going out late on pay day. Being a gas free mine, smoking was allowed, but at certain designated points usually where there are fresh air, we called it a vent flow. The charging up with explosive was completed, but for only the remaining holes to be drilled by the "late" machine operator. Above him sat the team leader waiting. In his hand was the igniter cord, having connected up all the panels charged holes, he lit a match to light a "zoll" or hand made cigarette. On lighting it the match accidentally came into contact with the igniter cord in his hand. Immediately it caught alight and a ball of bright red fire erupted. This ball of ferocious fire started its run op the face towards explosives and started to ignite it.

It was a fire from hell, flames advancing up the panel at great speed. The men reacted fast. The team leader was shouting in Fanagalo "balega balega" which means "run", it wasn't necessary because everybody was running and crawling away to safety anyway.

I also headed to the back area aiming to get behind a pack. The first shots went off with a deafening roar. Everything shook. The roof started falling in, slabs on either sides of me also fell. The body shaking concussions carried on. The earth shook. The blasted rocks directly from the blasted face came past me like deadly explosive rockets of death. I froze, my whole body froze and I went numb from fright, death at my doorstep.

After the shots stopped ,as if a war had ended, silence reigned, slowly I crawled out of my hiding place. Slowly so did the others, "shell shocked". After surveying the damage it was reported that no one was killed or injured. We would be the very few to come out of such a blasting accident unscathed, unhurt. Where there was support sticks there were only pieces left, where there was a rock drill machine, also pieces were left. We were lucky to be alive. Those working the other 9 panels above saw the smoke, heard the shots and ran. The loss of production was 10 faces not blasted. I was in deep trouble. The IOM was called in to hear the hearing, as it was a blasting accident, a mining law was broken. The TL was discharged and I was given a heavy fine of R10, donated to the orphanage. The incident would haunt me forever.

An underground fire: At the place of gold

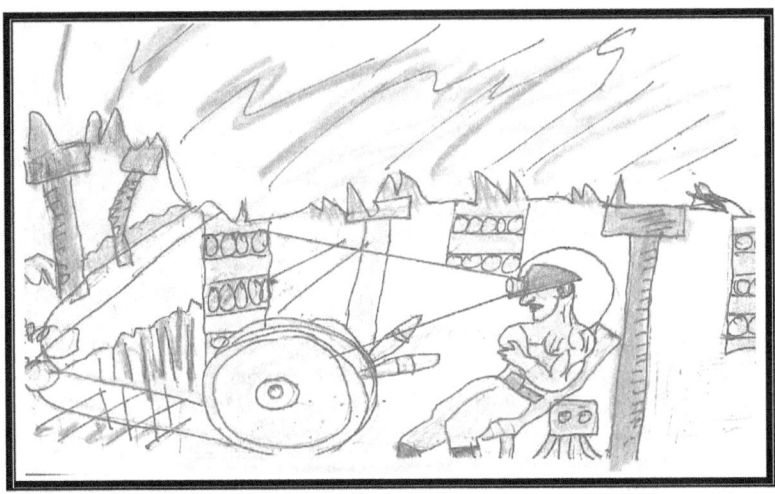

We read ,see and hear on television about underground mine fires. Those who know nothing about the working of a deep mine and have not been there and experienced it, will never know fully the implications to the psyche, and the pain of such a life threatening nightmare. To avoid this mine enforces very high standards and rules that must be taken to prevent these fires from happening. Just as in the strict enforcing of road safety with arrive alive campaign and so on, invariable accidents will occur. We all know over the years that over the Xmas period more that a 1000 road accidents occur resulting in such related car, bus, havoc wrecking deaths and injuries for life. The human error: factor? I survived this fiery out of hell underground fire experience.

The unexpected happened that dark steamy underground night. The very deep darkness suddenly became a daylight nightmare, the sound of crackling new wood burning furiously, a fire ball out of control. The night shift procedure on coming on shift was to check the safety which entails making sure the winches, ropes, scrapers, chains, snatch blocks and lastly the rigs in place and that they are properly secured and away from timber or support packs made of wood.

To explain further the cleaning process the winches, scrapers and ropes operate by bringing and carrying ore away from the face to a man made hole or tip. The scraper runs up and down the face, tipping the gold to the gully, from where it is pulled to the tip. Once all the before mentioned is in place the Team Leader signals by means of pulling a long wire, attached to an air signaling device. The scrapers can start moving up and own in rotation, one receiving the ore the other giving. The face winch driver was unfortunately a replacement from the day shift, doing a double shift being very tired and full of the Free State beer soon fell asleep behind the handles of the still rotating winch drums in full motion. To make it worse the team leader on the face also in a deep imbiber in strong alcohol fell soundly asleep like a new born. The top snatch block and rigs came loose. The moving ropes now fee cut into the top timber pack, knowing away up and down in a sawing fashion. High friction heat started. The ropes cut deeper onto the pack eating away, a combination of igniting grease on the rope. A mine fire had started; a tragedy was to occur, something that could have been avoided, human weakness apparent.

The support pack smoldered. The smoke from the fire grew denser, blacker. The once weak flickering fame grew bigger, stronger. It suddenly turned into a ferrous timber eating ball of red fiery destruction. The once deep blackness exploded into a Xmas tree from hell: with its bright light lighting up that total underground darkness. Those asleep, slept on, their deep breathing its sign. Smoke entered their nostrils, fright and consternation erupted, looking for water hoses, to put out the fire. They screamed hysterically. On the farm we would call people out of control like headless chickens .Luckily for me and the miner we had smelled the danger and were already in motion, pulling hoses and opening the taps for the water to stop the impending mine fire.

The strong ventilation flow had made matters worse, there were three packs burning, the flames darting and jumping from one pack to the next. The searing heat, pouring sweat, the blinded eyes, made it difficult to bring the now hot hoses to pint to the fiery flames. More hoses were pulled up, when six hoses were spurting all at once the fire started to subside, the whole area now thoroughly wet, muddy and sticky, the smell of teak wood smoke overpowering the area. Only half an hour ago all was well a life threatening event suddenly sprung up out of the pitch darkness, inferno, now just as it suddenly erupted it stopped. The sick pungent smell of burned timber was a blinding reminder of what just happened. It brought a sick stomach feeling. Men were lying down utterly exhausted, their chests in pain, breathing a mere choke, and we had won. The fire was out. The blackened ex-timber packs a grim reminder sight looking like skeletons burned out which will never burn again. Once the PROTO (fire control professionals) room on surface had picked up the signal of a mine fire the mine rescue teams were on there way, they were too late, their jobs were done by us.

The underground hair dresser 1980

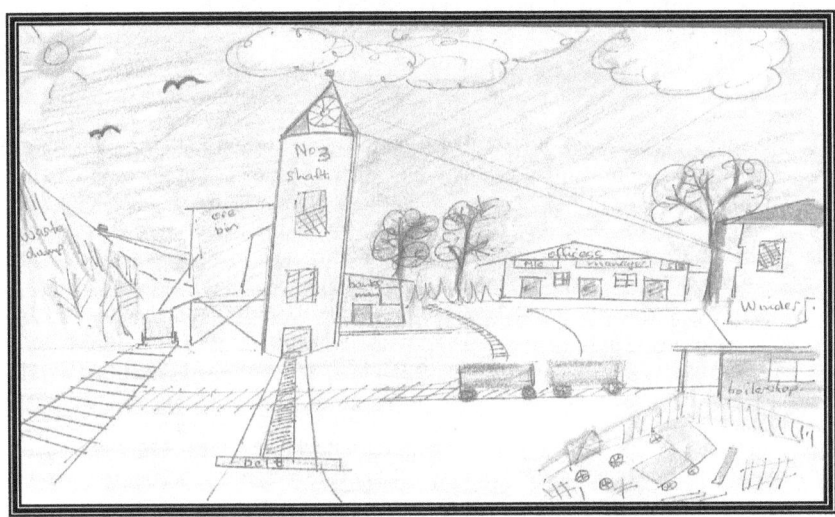

Alone stood the majestic mine shaft head in the African veld.

Through the lasing of the icy Free State winter it stood. In summer it was covered in tick mine dist blowing off the mine dumps, day becoming night. The structure was made of strengthened concrete, steel reinforcing and iron girders.

The shaft hole itself not round but oval in shape, this configuration proved to be more resistant to the earth's movement. On its great head were six huge turning wheels turning twenty four hours daily. These either pulled up the men working the mine, or the ore bearing ground from the deepest bowels of the earth. The ringing of the Banks man bells could be heard signaling to the Onsetter below to what level he should go to.

There were three shits in the 24 hours. The morning one provided the night sift with the necessary ore to tram to the shaft. The afternoon shift was put aside for the Engineering department. Their job was to check the shafts condition and do repairs. At the shaft bottom was usually an excessive amount of water, mud and rock fallen from the over-filled ore cage, you have to be on your toes if you worked there, ducking and diving, as you could hear the rock clanging it s way down as it struck the pipes in the shaft. Above the shaft bottom was the belt level. Here were situated many ore-pass openings with iron doors with strong handles to open them. At the end of the belt stood the bin in which, when the belt was in motion tipped the said ore, once the bin was full the bin controller would signal to the winch driver on surface to hoist it.

Of the three shifts I enjoyed the night shift, as a Shift-boss I had certain privileges, at my disposal was an office underground first aid bay store, and two phone, these connected to all the levels under my control and legal jurisdiction. My work entailed checking the safety of all working where miners were, the safe tramming of locos and hoppers, their click-clacking and warning hooter heard, the iron wheels grinding as they move through the maze of tunnels and haulages to tip their precious loads.

The different gangs would pass me as I sat at the store waiting place. Many different nationalities would greet me "How are you, Ntate Ramasimong?" They would chorus. One such a black man was a Shangaan hair-dresser. He always looked like a model on parade. He wore the non-regulatory white boots, white officials overall and white hard hat. No warning could change this attire. The gleaming white teeth could be seen in the gloom. Under this hard hat was another covering, a plastic "see-through". The shinny well combed hair glistening at the touch of cap lamp light. During the day he ran a booming hair-dressing business. He was also called "Mofie". During that time of the 1970's the gold mining industry was booming. All people black and white benefited, the gold fields of S.A. were a mass of workers, the churches full, the schools full, and businesses doing well.

My job on night shift was going safely my target met; suddenly the earth shook and gave a sight shudder. It was 4 am, the phones started ringing. That dreaded call, a fatal, a miner's nightmare.

A rock fall had occurred on level 44, the miner, my assistant and I quickly got on to the four wheeled bike and started pedaling like mad to the fallen in stope. On arriving there were, we trudged up the long 45° stair case to the top. Here the Team-leader in charge, Thabo greeted us, as is the custom, but was in a shocked state, his best friend the Winch driver, (Our "Mofie") was trapped under a pile of rock. We had come just in time to assist him in the rescue, he was already dead, his left arm missing. There was no evidence of blood loss. His torso from the neck down was crushed. We felt like puking, a friendly man a few hours before, now a corpse. My assistant shone his cap lamp on his head to examine further. There wasn't a scratch. The permed hair was still in tact, the black shiny Negroes curls glowing under the lamp light beam. Not a strand out of place. His face was in deep repose as if content, proving to all that even in death this underground hair-dresser guarded his precious hair up to the end, until death do us part!

Illegal miners: another look

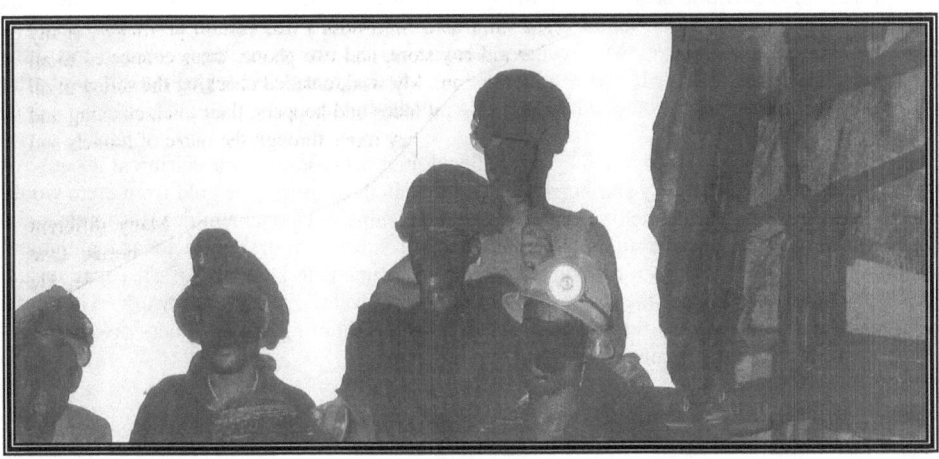

I read and heard about illegal miners on different mines in South Africa, but did not take notice as I had not seen any myself. On one of the shafts I worked on I was suddenly confronted with the problem. It came as a shock. On a certain shaft in the Goldfields, Welkom there must have been a 100 of them. I had to work night shift that week and on arriving at the waiting place, to my consternation there they were, 20 of them. Not showing that I was afraid I walked up to them. They greeted me with the traditional greeting of "Ntate" which means father. I asked them who they were and what they wanted. They answered they were hungry and were waiting for food provided by the gang coming up behind me in the rear. Making as if all was in order I sat down and waited, ignoring them. To my surprise the whole gang knew them and a chattering of bartering began. Many squashed loaves were pulled out of hats, shirts, trousers and overalls.

Chicken, polony and all type of groceries were exchanged for cash. Bread went for R20.00, a chicken for R50.00, the night shift miners were making a killing. In minutes they were all gone off to eat. A miner who did not look the other way and reported them would be taken care of. For example a white miner after been warned by them not to spy had his car stolen as warned. Beside that they stole his tools and sabotage his work place under ground, eventually he had to leave for another mine. I was more concerned for their safety and well being. The reason for this was that the more I came into contact with them the more horrified I became. First they did not look like human beings but like caged up animals in a Zoo. Staring eyes some were naked, some only had pants on. Most did not have a lamp to see, one out of 10 had to share a lamp. Some were reported to have AIDS, slowly dying curled up in pain. Those that did die were left on the station, a banks man picked the decaying body up and he would be on the pay roll.

Management was very worried. The company was losing tons of high grade ore from the faces. Those who did not work together with them were beaten. A shift boss was attacked, his genitals tied with rusting wire. Officials that were suspected of collaboration and found with money were fired. I was very careful to stay neutral. Many a morning security forces would round them up, send them back to their home lands, but in a week they would be back in full strength. The problem became out of control. Management were powerless, the more they got rid of them, the more they came back. Why? It was reported that the illegal miners were getting R30 000 after working for 6 months underground without seeing any daylight.

There families are starving at home they went illegal, in most cases to their detriment because of the diseases, solemnized, injury and horrifying death waited for them. The gold from them would make its way to illegal gold smelting plants in the town ships. Management decided to close the working shafts in that area overnight. A dispute had arisen between the contractors running them and the main parent company. Shutting down meant immediate stoppage of all cages to and from the work places because the electricity was put off no water pumps would work. The shafts were in effect flooded. Very few made it out to other neighboring shafts, others drowned in a sudden wave if oily water, a muted scream, a dreadful end.

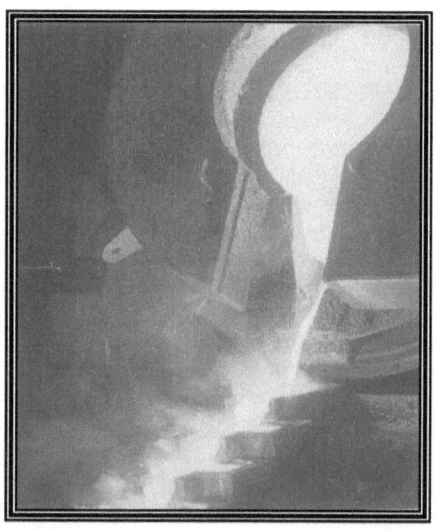

The Danger of an illegal diamond 1995

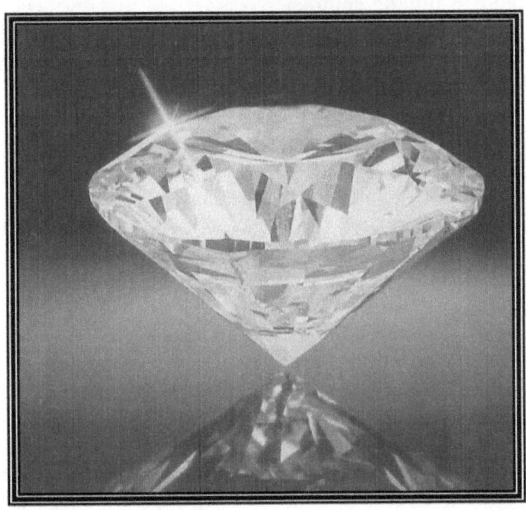

It is quite amusing that I never went out of my way to deal in elicit diamond dealing.

At the age of 50 I retired "officially from the mines. After working for 15 years as a Shift Boss at the No 3 President Brand Mine, Welkom, I called it a Day. The years was 1995 and most right wing whites were afraid of what would happen once Mandela came out of prison, I worked out that with the low taxes, there would not be a huge tax cut on the lump sum I would receive, but if I did stay on to the age of 60. I would lose half of it thereby losing double when a black president took over. I joined the stream of whites leaving, on the 03/08/1995, Martie, Angelique, Patrick and I went on a super holiday with the trailer packed with "pad-kos", hooked on the Toyota Cressida we headed for table Mountain and the great city called Cape Town.

We wined and dined at the best hotels, we toured the west coast and the Cape Point, saw Dagama's wooden cross and masses of baboons along the wayside. The mighty Indian Ocean and cold windy Atlantic meet is an eternal clash, steam spray, billowing into the sky day and night, day faster day. White seagulls flying about up and down, zigzagging diving onto the deep for tasty fish, shark fins seen through binoculars, making their silent and deadly stalk, looking for their prey, human or otherwise, imagining their razor sharp teeth, one bite and your leg is gone. Black and white dolphins parade up and down the rocks in the sun.

So we made our way to the East coast via Knysna, not knowing that one day our family would settle there. That night we arrived at Jeffery's Bay, we fell in love with the place. We bought two stands not on the beach but about half a kilometer from it, a short walking distance. On one of the stands we built a Igloo shaped house. To this day we love to go there and chill out and relax and forget. On getting back to Welkom, I was not prepared to go on real pension I had to get back to work searching for work through the local news papers. Looking for something different and exiting, I eventually found work in an area I had not worked before Kimberley.

The Big hole in the middle of town, there coca-pans sitting on its edge full of make believe diamonds, too many to count. A mining contractor was waiting for me. He promised me work on a nearby diamond mine. I was thrilled, having worked on coal and gold but not diamond. It was a challenge. We arrived as they say in Afrikaans in the "boendoe". The interview went well I being actually over qualified, being ranked as a shift boss and mine captain.

The work offer was for a miner, but I accepted the post. With a shake of hands, the new bosses showed me where I would stay. My new abode was a small caravan, next to a tree. Along side the tree was a small ablution block, a kitchen, toilet a sitting room and two bedrooms. These were already occupied by an Electrician and Boiler maker, so I was given the lone caravan under the tree. Walking distance from the sleeping quarters was the mine. Its officials to one side, small shaft head, with a winch. From this extend the important continuo's belt and plant to sort out the diamonds coming out of the mine.

The mode of transport to get to the underground workings was called "kibble". Five people were packed into it and with the required "ring" of the signaling device "clocks" or bells they were called, you would descent to the deep darkness. Slowly descending there were different levels or stations. Here the kibble would stop those getting off would do so. One ring would denote stop but you had to get out quickly on that level to do so. Once the winding engine driver receives the call, he stops until all have got out. A signal is given to raise the iron bucket to surface to fetch the rest of the crew.

Walking to the area where the diamonds were mined was a surprise to me. I was used to a large spacious tunnel or haulages these were small and half the size of those in the gold mines. One other surprise waited for me. I was used to a reef horizon, where the gold was lying usually at a degree of between 10° to 30°, here I found the face at an 90°angle, perpendicular, straight up, to mark off the holes to be drilled by the machine operators, one had to crawl and balance yourself precariously on sticks and gum planks attached or hit onto the side of the excavation.

Falling would mean a day or two in hospital. Doing the actual marking off with an aerosol red, you would start at the top, after making safe, barring with a pinch bar, the diamond area would now be ready for marking off. A stout manila rope would be tightly wound around your waist and as you marked off, you would be lowered slowly downwards. Once having completed this tenuous job you would escape the falling rock of the machine operator about to drill. At the end of the shift once the miner that me, has charged up the entire drilled hole you connect up and by means of a small machine called a blaster, you would blast the 30 odd holes. The diamonds would go into an ore pass situated below the said 90° face. The following shift would then draw the diamond bearing ore by coca-pan, from there to surface via the station ore pass.

I enjoyed working there the bosses amicable and friendly, the workers, the one half searched for illegal diamond the other "officially" working the work they were supposed to do the stolen diamonds were a huge bonus for the workers. We would see black a Mercedes arriving at the black hotels to buy these precious stones. Being caught meant arrest and a non negotiable prison stay.

One night I heard a soft knock on the caravan window. It was an illicit diamond dealer who I had repeatedly refused to accommodate. Through the opening of the window he pushed through a large brown envelope. Inside was one big brown precious diamond. I was shocked, caught and it would be the end of me. Hiding it under the bunker, I went to work, a troubled man, I wasn't a thief and would not start to be one now. Unfortunately the crook was waiting for me underground. I knew him well, the miners assistant. He asked me to meet a go between that night and he would take me to an isolated farm where the deals were done. I refused. A number of his friends appeared out of a cross-cut threatening me with my life. Forced to agree under this unexpected life threatening situation, I listened to their instructions.

At 2 am that morning, with the "agent" we arrived at the farm, a single large black Mercedes was standing outside of the home-stead. Shaking in my boots I walked in warily. At the head of a long table sat a very fat white man, a smirk on his face. His huge body guard sat a small distance away, watching intently for any aggressive action from me. "You are new to the game, he asked?" "Yes" I trembled, taking out the precious stone, the money to be halved between me and my tormentors back a the mine waiting- half a million rand was a lot of money, with it I could go and retire permanently at the coast. "fatty" had a number of ways to test whether it was an valid diamond or not, I sat there hell-shocked this was not my cup to tea, I was cohered to be here never the less I was counting the piles of money before it was given.

My Mother a teacher always said" Don't count the eggs before they are hatched" true words never spoken, with a start fatty threw me the diamond back, the gun man going for his 45 magnum, I nearly fell back off the stool with fright. "I will give you R10 for this shit, you wasted my time, fuck off or my friend will shoot you". Now trembling, I asked him what was wrong, "you have been had" he answered "What will I tell those who sent me" I answered. "That is your problem" He roared, "Now Go!"

The gun was pointing at me, I was a dead man, whether I went back or not, those waiting wanted the cut of the million. Staggering to the Toyota, the "go between" looking grim, I explained to him, that the fantastic diamond was in fact a piece of worth less shit, rock. I trembled putting, the envelope into his hands, "we are both dead" he mumbled. "Pack your bags when we get back, I will fetch mine at the hostel, the dealers will not believe us, we have to make a get away tonight, otherwise tomorrow we are dead meat" Back at the caravan I quickly reversed the car close to the door, I quickly packed my clothes, pots and pans. I left quickly, there wasn't time, and my life was in danger.

Was one of the Smugglers watching me? Would I get home safely? With spinning wheels, I drove like a mad man back to Welkom never to return.

The unforeseen: The mine accident

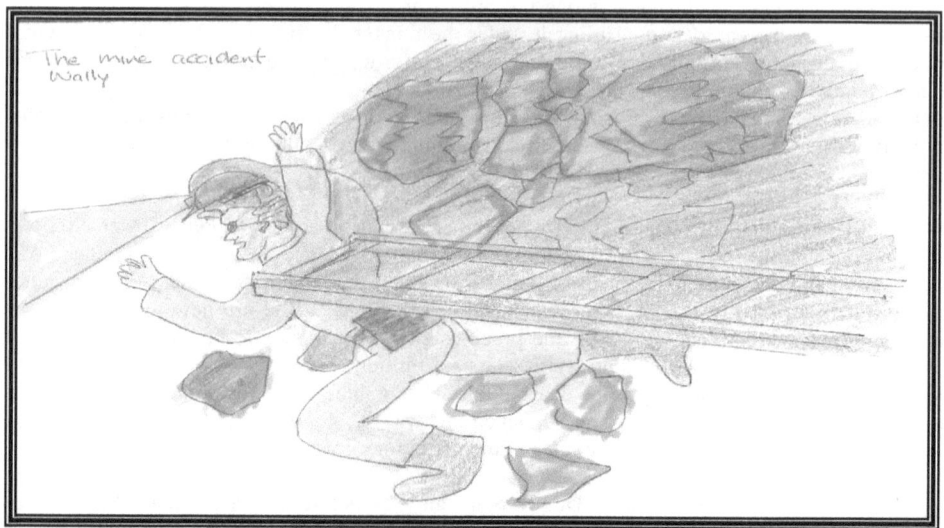

On a certain day the "Big Wheel" turned against me. The unforeseen happened. Unknown forces struck. My first mine accident happened, striking suddenly. The dark tunnels became darker; the fear of injury had arrived in the reality. My safe world came crashing down. While inspecting the workings in haulage as a Mine Overseer, I watched a scraped go back and forth scraping stuff to a ramp into a waiting hopper which would be tipped into the ore pass, from there up the shaft to the gold plant. The unthinkable suddenly happened, as light earth tremor occurred. An avalanche of loose rock came rushing down from all sides. I was in the middle, the wrong place at the wrong time. There was a thick cloud of dust, I could see nothing.

A great weight struck my waist, a terrible pain never before experienced overcome me. I fell heavily to the ground, pinned flat like a rat in a trap screaming. A hub rail switch was lying on top of me, it weight two tons. A trap of steel immovable the pain was the pain was terrible, a shattered pelvis. Like a jig-saw puzzle to be put together again. I calmly put my spectacles in my top pocket. Help was on its way. Luckily my Team leader David who I had promoted was nearby. On seeing the accident from a distance rushed at great speed with his gang to assist me. It took ten men to lift the steel switch off me using mine poles for leverage to free me from the mountain of loose rock. They had to lash with shovels and pinch bars to free me.

Once out on the waiting stretcher. Unfortunately they could not take off my overall. My right pelvis socket joint was dislocated, when moved I screamed, shocked they did not know what to do next. Their "Ramasemong" was by dying a frightful death in front of them. David my life saver, the leader took over, slowly they picked me up, lowered me on the stretcher. I was now unconscious a broken doll a limp thing. The cage came after the urgent phone call to surface. The ambulance had arrived, the wailing of its siren heard. After a morphine injection I was rushed of to I.C.U. Opperheimer Hospital. The shock to my body caused my lungs to collapse. I went into a coma. For two weeks my life hung on a thread. The Doctors were skeptical of my recovery. Shocked, my family was stunned. My ageing mother was rushed from Margate, fearing the worst, her eldest son was dying. Prayers were offered. The priest was called, the matter was serious, and a life had to be saved, extrimunction, a prayer for the dying.

The body damaged:
1. Assessment, broken pelvis in six places, it was shut closed like a book
2. Dislocated pelvis joints.
3. A ruptured stomach
4. A ruptured bladder
5. Lungs full of fine mine gold dust.
6. Double Pneumonia

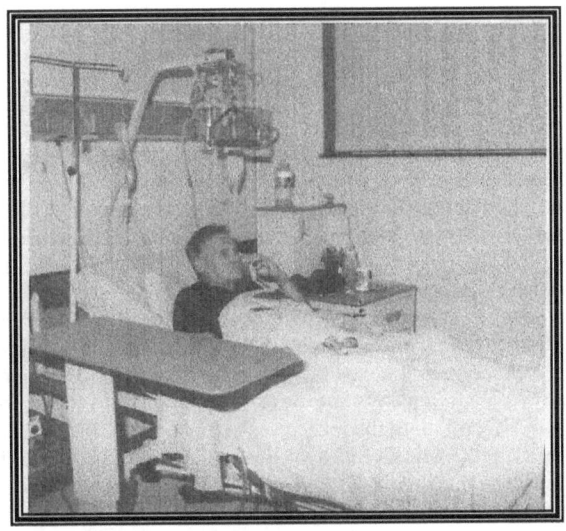

Trembling Jelly

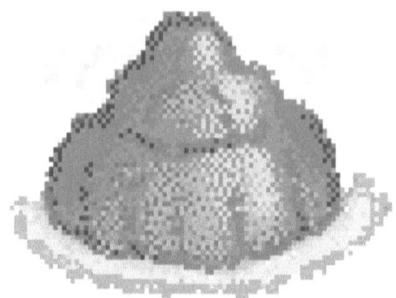

Trauma center unit

The day light and night, light and night were the same, day and night, night no difference. I never knew what time of day it was, or what day, week or month. The minutes, hours, weeks ticked slowly by, but the pain and suffering permiated the atmosphere. The doctors and nurses at their posts, helping, studying charts, taking temperatures, examining patients.

Why was I there? It was the cause of a mine accident, broken, cracked, splintered pelvis, ruptured bowls and bladder. Through my veins coursed a pain reliever called morphine, a narcotic opium. My thoughts were those of a man in a deep dream, a kaleidoscope of colors flashing past the inner eyes looking: the past rushing away like a flooded river in full spate. My family members each one parading past, some were smiling, others I trying to tell them to go a different way, a safer way. Don't go to the left go to the right. I was floating around the hospital, listening to the remarks of the Doctors. My own life was hanging by a thin thread. They were worried "Will Gird pull through, or will we lose him?" What alternative are there? Check the charts, his blood content, too much iron or magnesium. A long row of blood ingredients, check, we must not lose him, it also depends on his will to fight to survive, a mitigating factor in my favor. Hope against hope and faith.
Martie my loving wife was always there for me, exhorting me to get better soon.

I was worried about her as, she looked the picture of forlornness and sadness, was she coping with out me, looking after Angelique in Matric and Patrick in standard one, Lillian, Hannes and Walter how were they coping? Charlotte heavy with her first pregnancy, Quintin as security guard lying in the bushes with Monastery the Alsatian, was he safe from those intended burglars of mine property. My two brothers Aussie in New Zealand in the biting snow, Mike his obsession with money and status. Can he see further that those demigods, I pray for him to get out of that false tightening web. What about my own soul? Will my own sins send me to hell? I was high on drugs; I waited for the next shot of morphine, a return to the safe haven of the dream world.

Time passed by my body shriveling from 90kg of hard exercised muscle to a worm's weight. Muscles out of order but the heart, lungs and inner organs functioning on, unstoppable, the great sprit of God was watching. On one occasion I thought it was time, time to die. Two patients next to me did die within minutes of each other. I heard the thump, thump of the Doctors hammering on their hearts, resuscitating them to no avail. "I have done everything possible, but now he is gone" I heard the other Doctor sighing in resignation "Go to the next patient" I was terrified, was it me? Was I the next one? I trembled and shacked. Their conversation receded into the distance; I was safe for the time being.

My spirits drooped I became chronically depressed. I asked Martie to contact a physiatrists, I don't want to die yet! With out me knowing it she was on her way. One very dark night I felt a very soft touch. It was a saving hand a hand of hope, there were others beside me. A soft voice out of that darkness said "how are you? You will get through and get better soon, you have what it takes, your strong faith, hope and love for others well beings will pull you through, she continue softly, whispering in my ear. It was like giving me water just before collapsing in the fiery hot desert sand in the Sahara desert. I thought it was a dream, hallucinations! Unexplained, the next day I was on the way to recovery. Later I was told the loving Psychiatrist visited me!

It was close to a month, 30 days with out eating. Intravenously yes, solids no, after many operations during that time it was also time to get better and well, that "worm" not a man had to get back on his feet. He wasn't made to lie on his back, naked. After much deliberation the powers in charge decided to take the drips off, the morphine away and the intravenous food. "Tomorrow you will eat" the doctor said to me happily. I was ecstatic. The next morning true to promises the food came. A big plate of putu pap with a large egg on top of it arrived. "Eat: ordered the male nurse, I was dumb founded, I could not eat solid foods after 31 days of watery foods "No" I said "There must be a mistake, fetch me the Doctor now.

On arriving the said doctor was horrified; "bring him some jelly" he thundered. Attracted by this commotion the rest of the staff come and stood around the bed of the Ramasong, knowing my Sotho name by now. This crowd now stood expectantly waiting for me to eat. All eyes were on me, the make nurse now contrite gave me the jelly. In one hand I held the tea spoon, in the other the small plate of jelly. Dipping the spoon hesitantly into the jelly my whole body was shaking from the effort "Come on" screamed the expectant crowd, "Eat" they roared. Slowly, shakily tremblingly the spoon and jelly approached my mouth, teeth chattering and clicking.

Shaking like a leaf a half of a teaspoon full went in my first food, manna out of heaven, saving grace, a miracle!

Yes, I was stronger and better.

That trembling jelly saved my life.

Chapter 2
Early years

Chapter 2   Early years

Looking from an eye of an eagle

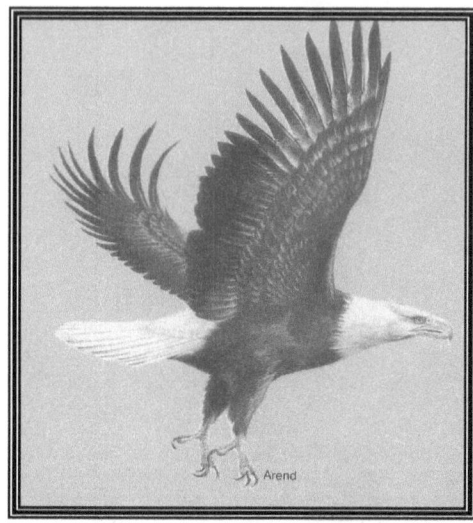

Looking from an eye of an eagle from far in the bright blue sky you could see the Easter Free State topography a landscape stretching and undulating with hills and mountains increasing in mass and number as they multiplied towards the higher ranger of Lesotho.

Our story begins in this area of small mountains and small "koppies". These had beautifully descriptive names such as "hoepel rok", the shape of a yester year fashionable dress of Old Dutch descent. "Mensvretersberg", a mountain feared only by rumor of its past cannibal history. A place where you were eaten alive in a pot of local herbs and boiling steaming water, a scream heard, or a human "braai". True or false we children were terrified even to look in the direction of that cursed place.

Another even more spectacular mountain with a strongly fittingly name given by the locals was Thaba Nchu because when it rained, looking through the mist gloom the huge masses of granite rock turned blackish in colour.

The water borne wind came from the South twisting around those granite masses bringing with it much needed rain, also bringing the terrible drought to a merciful end. This saturated sea of water, the Eastern Free State earth and foliage, brown grass absorbed and drank with a great relish. The natives thanked their gods, the Boers their God of their bible.

Hordes of sandy brown coloured Afrikaner Cattle had their backs to the driving wind and icy rain. A few Basotho ponies stood resolutely under a copse of willow tree next to a now strongly flowing stream. A lonely hill or koppie named "Rekoy" was a witness to a simple birth of a white European Squalling red faced English boy. The other witnesses were the black and white midwives and helpers at 4 o'clock that morning.

Glamorgan "Thaba Nchu"

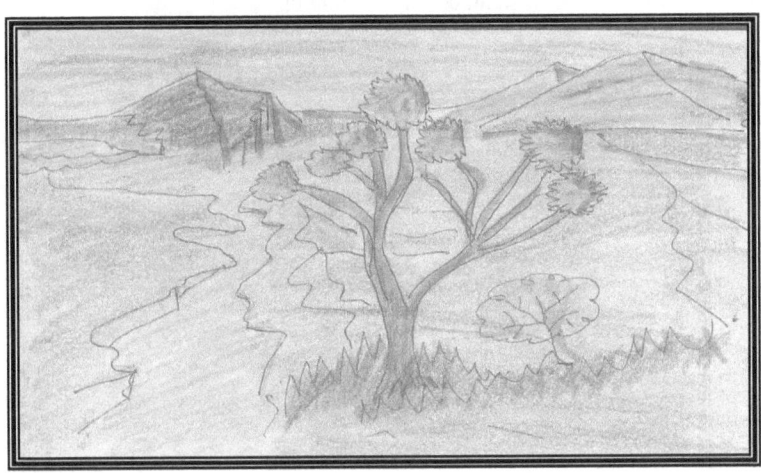

The storm had abated the sun rays becoming a soft glow in the east, showing the house and surrounding area to be awash. It was a sign of good fortune said the helpers to my smiling mother, looking at her new born. She would call him Walter, but the farm workers would gibe the name "Ramasenmong" the father of the fields. Two brothers would follow after me, Austin and Michael, both fair skinned, strong and energetic.

This happened just after World War 2 and according to my mother my dad came back a changed man. He went away to the war a friendly mild farmer; he came back with an unsettled state of mind. He had been shot at, his friends blown up next to him. After four years if hell, fighting in many countries including Germany and Italy he was never the same, but a man of great faith. His duty was to bring up children in the faith. We settled down at a place called Brandsdrift, the center of a rural farming community.

Here the Gird family of five grew up happily. Around our homestead grew many kinds of trees especially blue gums reportedly imported from Australia, all very high and straight. The early morning were the most memorable because of being awakened by hundreds of different kinds of bird life living in the trees around the house. In spring swallows came in their thousands, with chirping and chitterling mass made their nests at the rivers under bridges. These nests were made of clay, twigs and pieces of grass. My mother was my first teacher at home and then at school, my dad providing the chicken destined for our table, "finger licking good". For sport he played at the prestigious Westminister golf club.

A few unusual things to remember there were the greens. They were covered with a thin layer of gray coloured sand, not river sand but sand. This sand was pulled level by means of a very wide sacking pole. The specialized person was not seen as a farmer but a professional in his field. Those having just played a hole had to automatically level the playing field.

The other memory jogger was the long- drop toilet with two toilet seats one small the other larger, but to sit there and look down to the murky depths with spiders and all, this all made us very scared. There were stories of small children falling in.

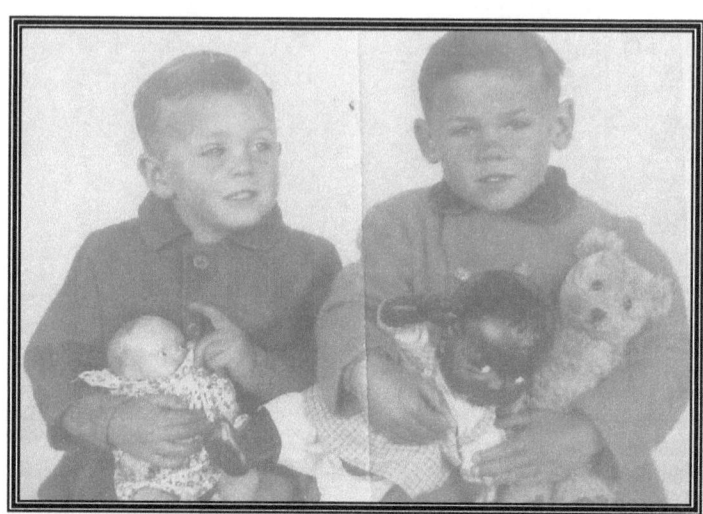

Austin and Walter at Thaba Nchu

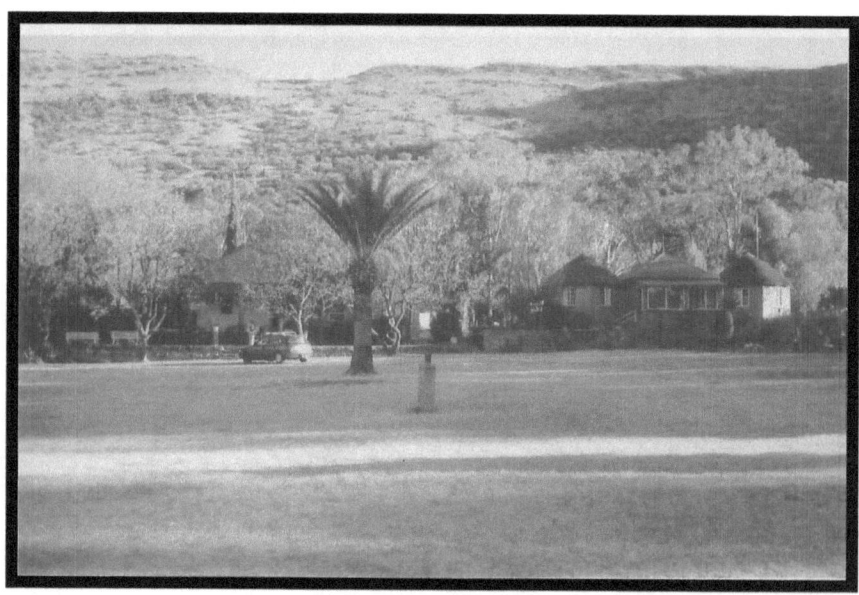

Glamorgan

Masepa

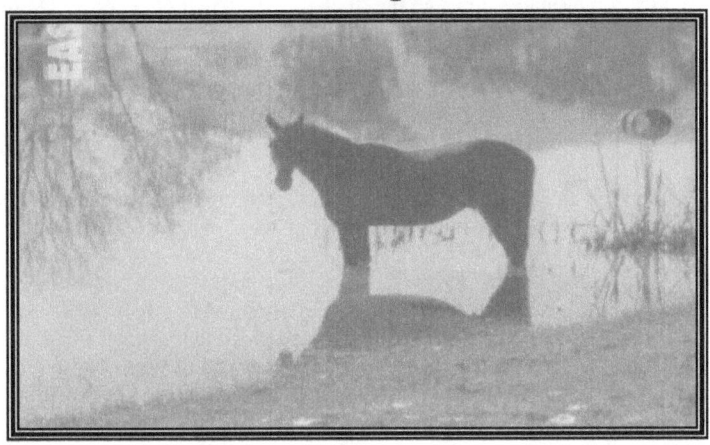

Masepa was a Basotho horse name, a derogatory word in the Sotho language for some one being "full of shit". He, a stallion, wild, untamable, having grown up on the mountain with out restraint of human domination, was a freedom fighter not to be saddled. He had a strong mind of his own. His spirit was that of the wild quagga, or zebra, found in the Bloemfontein area. He was part of the bush, and rolling hills, of the Easter Free State. It was rumored by the black folk in that place that this scraggly horse was sired between a lonesome normal farm stallion and a tame zebra. A first! The white farmers did not believe this superstition story, but one of them while hunting did see him fleetingly. He reported seeing the rays of the sun slanting on his hind quarters showing diagonal black and faded stripes down those flanks, muscles rolling and rippling, a ball of energy ready to gallop at moments notice, or at the sound of a crack of a twig broken in avertedly by a human foot.

Where this free animal lived was on a farm called Glamorgan, a name reaching back to its first owners the Morgans, they were of Welsh extraction, hence the Welsh name. At the rear of the two home steads next to each other, one a thatched roof the other zinc was and is Thaba Nchu Mountain. There those granite sand stone bulges of rock and cliffs, stood when the foul weather abated and the mist cleared, those colours turned a grey black, hence the name black mountain.

The herds men on that farm from time to time herded up all the "strays roaming there, among these were many African cattle reddish in colour extracts of those mighty Boer ox wagons, now a product seen all over South Africa's landscape, a sturdy ox used for plowing the maize fields. Among this capture were also she goat and Billy goats who would rush at you at any sign of antagonism, stray cows, and sheep and of course the hero of our story, Masepa among them.

The farmer in charge even up to this day is that mighty man of 2 meters, them now a bent gnarled man on crutches, a man who was feared then, and his boxing knocks bent and cracked a testomy to discipline, enforced. Besides being strong he was a outstanding consiour of the siring, and the upgrading of Merino sheep for the high value of their white wool. He could count 300 of them at high speed as they came out of the open gate in two or three at a time. As young boys it was our greatest pleasure to visit him at Glamorgan, I was 10 at the time. After the formalities of greeting him, Rilly our aunt, Ann, and Joy our close cousins, we headed for the mountain side. After sight seeing and walking on the dam wall lined with willow trees and bushes we headed back down to the two home stead's, through the thick forest of high blue gums. On the verandah we all had the pleasure of having tea, muffins and scones, dripping with fresh cream. The exquisite China set was used. The cups were hand painted showing Chinese figures, the edges lined with a rim of gold. These figures were painted in blue. One figure was a man on a ski- paddle in one hand, the other waving to his love who had turned into a swallow and was flying away.

A foreman came up to the gathering, with great humility, with hat in hand reported the rounding up of those motley lot of animals found on the mountain side. Klaas gave me a direct challenging look inviting me to come, his strong white teeth glinting, his goatee beard pointed and bobbing, with the smile. I was his favourite, besides knowing his language, always had a piece of rolled tobacco for him from my dad's store at Brandsdrift where we lived. The Girds there, the Higgses at Glamorgan. Aussie came with. We arrived at the stables and were surprised to see how many different strays had been rounded up. Around these run away animals was a wall built of hand cut sand stone, neatly built by long gone crafts man. The rocks transported by ox wagon, twenty African oxen pulling the tonnage, the long leather whips resounding crack echoing through the line of cliffs and boulders high above on that black mountain. What caught the eyes of Aussie and my self was the wild horse, Masepa. The herdsman and all the boys had tried to ride him bare back, all falling off.

He could not stand still for a minute his muscled legs twitching as he stamped his hooves, in irritation at his untimely and unasked for capture. The blacks encircling him tried to keep him calm for the small "morena" to try his luck at a ride and expected fall into the dirt and manure. "Throw the lasso over his head" I commanded. Momentarily still, the mongrel horse glared at me, mad eyes rolling, the whites showing. Taking a running leap I landed squarely on his back, rough and thorny. Luckily the bridle and reins were already on, so with one hand on the sandy mattered hair the other holding onto the leather for dear life away we went, hooves pounding the foot path. I was on a runaway horse, out of control, the highly defied fore quads, legs run in tandem to each other. I was floating, not in a canter motion, but flying wildly effortlessly the legs rotating, between my bunched tightly holding legs, I was slipping on the strong slimy horse covered in sweat. Tail flying, main on one end, Masepa was enjoying himself with his game of death, I was not. On reaching the out most frontier of the farm, he swerved to the right at an angle, towards the road running from the main on to Bloem. Through bush and sloot we traveled, turning again now into the road back to the home stead's. All I could see were the rows of trees planted in lines flashing past; he was heading back to the "kraal" and slowing down, until he went into a canter. At the kraal was a crowed waiting cheering me along.

At first apprehensive, now glad to see me back safe and so sound on Masepa's back on passing the gate with our further ado, our wild friend went to the 45 gallon trough of spring water and with bent neck drunk in long slurps to his full. Off I jumped now very groggily from that aggressive exertion; it was the horse ride of my life, a first for Masepa!

I write this story for Austin my brother, who urged me to do so.

"Hoot" the Owl
The Eastern Free State

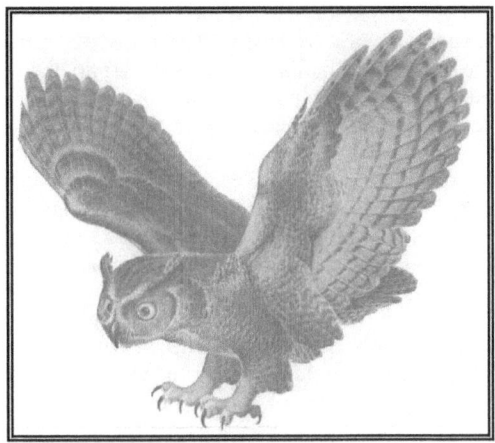

In his young life he was very independent and self reliant. Sitting in the dark, high above the ground, alone, perched on a gum tree's branch. The oozing gum a glued to his claws, slightly, irritatingly because it would hinder his sudden attack on his prey below. It was dead of night, its hour just past, struck. The echo's of his mournful hooting resounding the muffled way in the forest enclosure. An early feeling was felt, a feeling of the unknown haunting sound.

Unknown to our hero the owl, high above in the heavens slow drifting light flaky snow was coming off the clouds and south wind. The winter was heralded in! The first snow always dropped far to the south, the Western Cape, the Swartberg. From there it was off loaded up to the great "dragon" mountain, the Drakensberg range. Closer to home the Malutis were now white capped, the thin wind whipping layers off, fortunately our bird friend and neighbours farm hands were in warm mud huts and the main home stead was partially protected and enclosed by a ridge of boulders. Thaba Nchu or Black Mountain in its protecting arms circle, they sat. This farm was named Glamorgan, of past Welsh extraction, from generation to generation.

Thaba Nuch's great granite boulders were seen to be glistening with fresh just fallen snow. As the winds broke up the Cumulus above, it was as if a pale reflection was seen of that cold ball of light far into the opening heavens, the moon. The snow cracked and hardened a severe warning to plant life in the morning. The most striking feature of our hooter owl was his eyes. They were round, wide, large and set to face foreword. Reeling through the gloom, he rotated his head slightly from side to side, all tension and concentration. Each eye was encircled with a ring of feathers as it were giving him a "wise" look. Two on the head tufts were seen as if were ears, bur were not.

His true hearing was hidden, but was exceptionally keen. To enable him to swoop most silently and quickly, his feathers were soft and aerodynamic. Highly muscled quads gave him that impetus for sudden action. His feathery markings were beautiful, but in statue smaller than his counter parts, the owl eyeing the ground below he noticed a slight movement. Was it a succulent mouse below the frosty level? Being an African predator, he was disciplined and patient. That was the first part of his hunting skills the second part, steely determination!

It was late. He was hungry, hooded eyes focused, slits, not closed, or asleep. A ball of concentration, nerves on edge. Suddenly in a bush nearby a commotion erupted, a unexpected sound of snapping and breaking twigs were heard. A sparrow was ruffling its feathers because of the cold and effort to get the blood running to get warm. Angry the owl flapped his wings in disgust, his focus momentarily put off. Soon he was back on his vigil, as a Free State Cheetah as it were, stalking his kill, but not moving a sinued muscle.

His hypnotic gaze caught sight of a pair of red eyes and a black nozzle. The red eyes were from the smarting berg wind, they belonged to a fat rat. He squealed from the pain of the ice. It was the opening; the hoot owl was looking for a partially blinding fat rat. Tipping forward, allowing his weight and earths gravity to do the work, he let go of the branch.

He fell like a heavy rock on to the unsuspecting prey. He descended at great speed, a shadowy flash of power. A swoop onto a kill, talents outstretched, vice like, to be applied. Bones were crushed to a pulp. The fat rat never saw him coming, or the light of morning. For the owl he was another statistic. From the branch where he sat, to the ground and back again, took a matter of seconds.

The graceful motion was done in a wide arc, flowing from one point to the next objective achieved. With a giant swallow he gulped in his meal. The aftermath of this blood lust brought on a gleeful delight, a happy flapping of his wings.

To the east the warmer sun ball was creeping, out, it was time for the day's awaited sleep. Those silted eyes closed, dozing. Could you hear him snoring? Was it the sound of the leaves ruselling or the crunching sound of the swaying tree trunk?

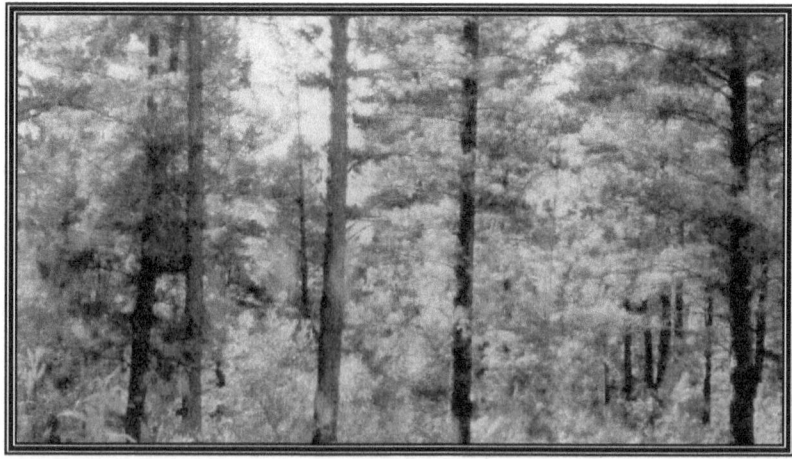

Brandsdrift 1950

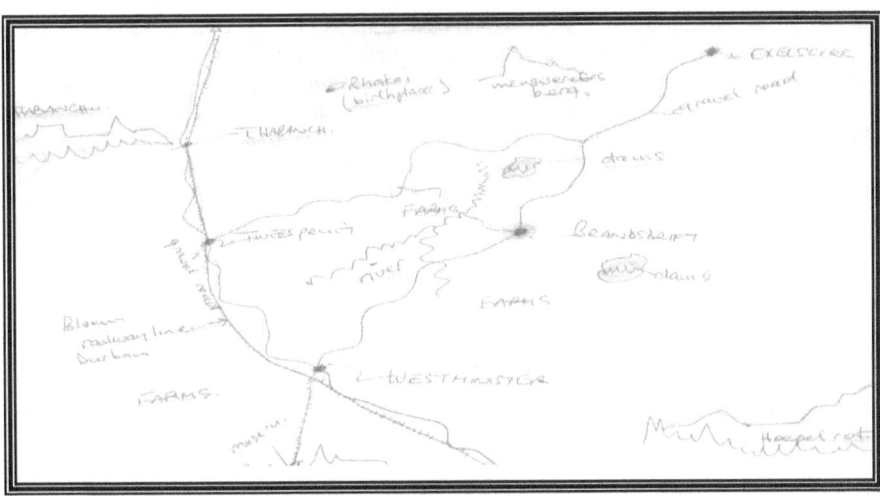

In the middle, the tranquil river made two pronged forks. Across these two points were straddled two low level bridges. In the winter there was no problem with the water flow. The water was being cold and icy floating on it many pieces of broken up ice melting in the winter sun. In some places where there were many weeds the ice blocks struggled to go with the flow. The sniping wind always came from the Lesotho Maluties, not far to the east.

The summer months were hot, if it did not rain. The Free State's wide open spaces where known for their infamous explosive electrical storms. These appeared out of the South causing havoc. When it became suddenly dark as it were night it became deadly quiet, trouble was near. The rule of thumb was first you see the flashing forked lightning, and then you hear the rumbling thunder afar. If and when the storm struck without warning on top of you, your blood turned to ice. The ringing of the thunder in your ears, the fright when suddenly a nearby Gum tree is struck down, its smoldering smell when grass alights, the flames flicker, but die out just as quickly in the pitch darkness and the pouring rain dowsing it. I loved to listen to the rain drops lash against the corrugated iron slopping green painted roof. It was like music and reminded me of the train wheels clack ting over the rails. The following morning was always deceptively quiet, trying to hide as it were, the violence of the night before. The local farmer would look and search for missing lambs or run away Afrikaner oxen. Hopefully the dirt roads were in tack, but in most cases what reminded was a sloot where the road should have been.

Hopefully his maze crop had got its quota of required water and not stop growing until its height of 2m was reached, the Basotho dwellings were usually hit the worst. Being made of mud and cow dung as cement they were no match against the elements. The rushing water would eat its way at the base of the hut; it would collapse like a pack of cards, a muddy mess. One reason for these huts falling so quickly was their proximity to the river. Water would not have to be carried far. On television you see many who build there shanties right next to the Vaal river, in dry consequences. The more strongly Boer homesteads would only have sprung a roof leak. The farmer would jovially say to his wife "Die dak lek gaan haal 'n emmer my vrou" answering she would say "Jou gat my skat, doen dit self" (The roof is leaking my wife go and fetch a bucket: No! Do it yourself)

Outside the stone building sheep or oxen would have gone astray. The search was on for them to find. Roads made of gravel were just gone, where there was a road now there was none. The Ford tractor had to be fetched, with a home made scraper in tow. A new one was started. The air after the storm was clear and fresh. In the hazy distance were the foothills of the great Maluties, there colour dimly fading from a true blue to a hazel green. We small boys loved to play in the dams of muddy water, making boats made of bamboo we would watch them disappear down the sloot, in the after math of the storm. Aussie reminded me of a hippo with his white posterior just above the waterline. Mike just starting to talk, his mop of magnificent fair hair bobbing up and down, his face muddy, teeth shining were laughing with delight. My Dad was not as happy as his Ford V-8 had got stuck. It's back driven wheels having sunk it further in to the mire. His customers were waiting impatiently at his shop door. Mr. Du Toit our land lord was obliging enough to pull out the bakkie with a span of Afrikaner oxen, their muscles straining and bulding.

The V-8 came out with a pop, covered in slimy mud. Those were the good old days. Today we can only reminisces on the past, smiling.

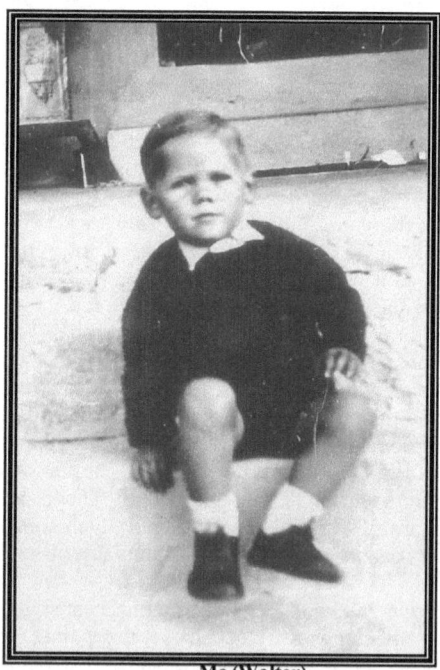

Me (Walter)

Condensed Milk

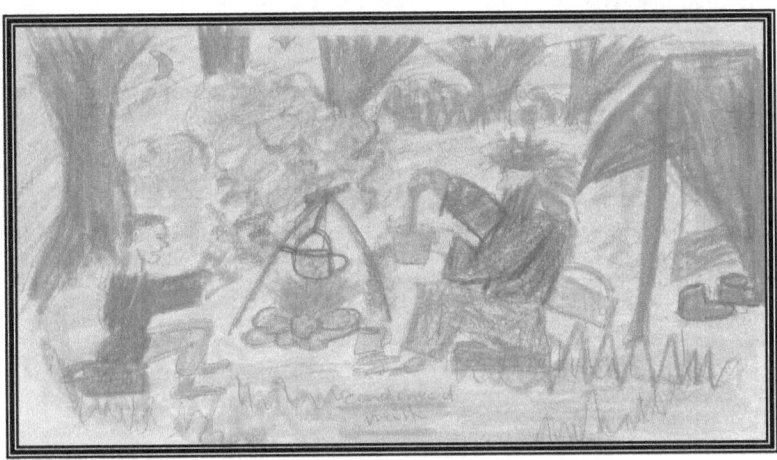

Bransdrift was a tranquil place to be, if you wanted quiet and peace. The quietness was to me as breathing. The other natural sounds were those of our farm life the crowing cock the mooing cows, the horses neighing. These were sounds I grew up with not really realizing that there were other disturbing sounds else where.

Unexpectedly I would find out sooner that I thought we were on the way to the great city of Johannesburg. We arrived after many uncomfortable hours on the road at Edenvale. Here my uncle Ralf and aunt Beryl lived. Ralf was an ex-army soldier and ex-prisoner of war, greatly traumatized; both were always smiling and friendly towards us boys. Our three girl cousins were always giggling; we got nervous and always fled from them. Farm girls are more understandable. I could not sleep at night. The terrible sound of the sudden roar of a lorry growling past the bedroom window, the cars breaks and wheels screeching at the stop street were too much for a farm boy, suddenly thrown into that cesspool of noise.

Lying in bed I would wonder: Where were the night sounds of the owl hooting from a far staring out from its dark perch, the lambs searching from their mothers lost in the night? They were thirsty for mother's milk. I wanted to go home now. To make it worse, my nieces complained that we boys were unfriendly and unsociable. We didn't understand their language any way. May be it was our fault, so our appearance looked quiet funny, close cropped hair sticking out around the ears, long khaki brown shorts, then it could be understandable. Eventually we said our goodbyes and off we went back to the land we were used tom the Free State, the place of milk and honey, for us anyway.

On arrival back it did not take me long to see a difference. Across the gravel road from our house between the eucalyptus trees and thick bushes a gray wisp of unknown smoke was seen. On enquiring from the maid, Augustina she said it was a "pad-loper" camping. She had seen him when walking to her mud hut rear the river a mile away.

Intrigued by this unexpected visitor I was determined to visit him that night as my mother had already refused permission "No" she said "strangers are dangerous". I went any way. Just after sun down my parents liked to chat over a glass of wine, I went visiting. Creeping stealthily between the bushes towards the stranger in the gloom, he saw me first. "Wie is daar?" He called out gruffly. With some trepidation I took hold of the offered hand in greeting. His hand felt like rough sand paper. Switching to English he bade me welcome. In the gloom of the light fore I could just make out his outline. He had a long scraggly beard, a tooth missing in front and he stank like hell. His breath was that familiar wine smell, the same as that of my Dad when saying good night with a kiss after night prays. This mans friendliness was more overpowering that his unwashed smell. I liked him, a dark angel, telling me all about events and places exiting and new to me. Looking at my luminous had a numbers watch I bade my new friend goodbye. It was time to creep unnoticed back to my bed, luckily not in the house itself where I could be heard but in a veranda room.

My mother also being my first teacher at Westminster primary school noticed that I was not concentrating on my times-tables. She warned me in a stern manner that the cane could be used, to help me remember. To tell the truth my thoughts were else where. What roamed about in my head were all the stories told to me that night before. The wandering ghost mad man, of how he had conquered the wide world, steaming owner the stormy ocean as a mighty sailor. He had shot many terrible looking prates. He bad slept with bitches of all sizes and colours. Being a small boy I wondered why he slept with so many dogs, did he enjoy it?

On one unlucky night he got into a drunken brawl. Three coloured vagabonds attacked him, leaving him for dead. On waking he found himself in a white lighted hospital. Half the top of his head was missing, a jaggered hole. He was never the same again. Unable to get back onto his ship again, he was discharged inabscentia. The company pay master bade him farewell with a hand shake and $50, he felt rich. That night sitting next to him, the bent blackened kettle steaming, he had bad news for me. Anxiously, looking at me that black hole in the dark where his forehead was. I waited for him to tell me some more exiting stores. He stated by saying once he had money in his pocked he was free to go onto the road pointing northwards. The mighty gold mines of Johannesburg were waiting for him. He was going to be rich. He had actually got lost leaving the N1 by mistake and landed up at Brandsdrift inadvertently. He was also rested and would be on his way before sunrise the next morning.

I was heart broken; we were just starting to get to know each other. We were just starting to know each other and now he was leaving for good. Watching me in my forlornly state he offered me a peace pipe the way the Indians would have done, "I offer you the best man made coffee this side of the ocean" his voice quivering. He produced two bent, well used also backend coffee mugs. After making the coffee with grounded caffeine, boiling water he took out a tin of condensed milk. That was strange to me, as we only drank milk straight from the cow's, nice and fresh. Like a life ritual he commenced to pour a long stream out of that tin of whiter that white condensed milk. Stirring both mugs he watched me intently. "Drink" he commanded, "you will never taste coffee like this again". Stirring and blowing the steam a way I drank.

Never in my entire life had I tasted such coffee. The sweetness blew me away. The coffee must have had a magic drug in it. I sat mesmerized. Not wanting to leave so soon.

On coming back from school that next afternoon, I came to "dead mans door" as promised. His make-shift tent of torn army canvas was missing; all that was left were the cold coals, dead with water thrown over it. Blinking with tears away I noticed something flashing under a near by bush. It was the two holed condensed milk tin, empty.

Even up to this day I vividly remember that scalding hot coffee made of 100% condensed milk.

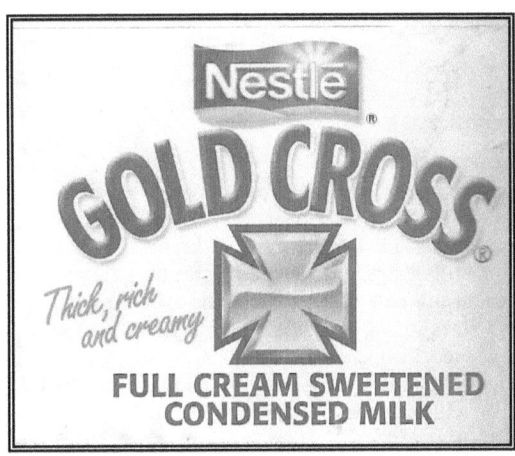

Chewing a snake's head

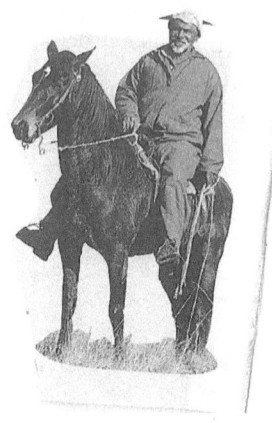 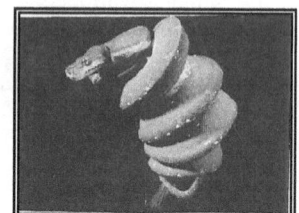

The adventure took place at Glamorgan farm below Thaba Nchu Mountain. At that time we were herding the cattle to dip them for tick fever. I was on the back of a Basotho pony moving them towards the narrow tailings for dipping. The "kraals" were made granite some blocks which even after 100 years still standing. Protruding from a pole was a hook I passed through the narrow gate. This caught my belt. The horse shied away leaving me suspended in the air. My uncle Buffy, a big and strong man, also had a bad day. He was attacked by a buck on heat. They said the buck was locked in one of the kraals when it happened. Up to today nobody knows what really happened. The buck did get way to its mate; my uncle did received injuries to his legs. Today he walks with crutches. I am sure he will deny the story, but my mother laughing told me the tale.

The great outdoor held a great fascination for me and my brothers. We had black friends who were sheep and cattle herders. We had many mock "battles". Standing in lines opposite each other across the steam we would shoot each other with "clay-lat". These were long thin braches stripped of bark and could bend easily to be able to shoot a ball of clay at the opponent. Smoking was not for me. Smoking dry horse or cow manure, wrapped in brown paper, make me sick for a week. I've never smoked again. An old black with a small pointed white beard in a Basotho pony used to greet me often at the trading store, always asking for a roll of tobacco. My answer was always no, because I never had money to buy it for him. In the "veld" were many dead mice or small snake. This I found and put a "ringkals" in an old news paper used at the shop. He arrived with his usual greeting of "Lekay?" How are you? With a wicked grin I gave him the "tobacco". He gave his thank you put it in his top picket and rode slowly away.

What happened a few miles way was told to me by my herder friends. They saw the old man chew the tobacco, but with a snakes head in his mouth, he gave a loud yell. His horse reared up and galloped way leaving him behind. My dad asked me later about the poor complaining man who wanted a tobacco refund I knew nothing, but hid away when I heard he came looking for me.

The Ghost

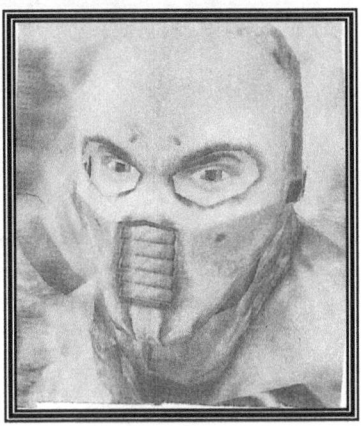

The trade store my father rented was on the farm of a Mr. van Wyk, who had a naughty son, always playing tricks on people. On dark night we were having supper as a family when we heard a loud knocking on the front door. We had no electricity and either used candles or gas lamps. I hurried to the front door with the candle, hot wax running onto my burning hand, the flame spluttering nearly going out. I opened the door. There stood a ghost, a grotesque maniac. I let out a terrified scream. My Dad came running at high speed to my rescue, a fist flew, a knuckle cracked. A muffled sound erupted when the perpetrator fell into the rose garden, the thorns pricking him. The "ghost" pleaded for mercy. It was the farmer's son. "Dit is ek Oom" he screamed. With a broken nose and split upper lip. His ghost mask shattered, his glasses smashed. He was a sorry sight to see that week, a blue swollen face. A boy dejected. On another occasion, his Dad sent him to fetch the maid servant who had mot completed cleaning the floor properly. On arriving at the stream where she was washing clothes, being of quick temper and very demanding, he ordered her to come immediately. She refused and would come later. He struck her on the forehead with his right fist. Partly stunned and falling and to stop her from collapsing on the ground she grabbed. Unfortunately for the farmer's son a part of his genitals, was hanging out. She held fast onto the left one. She tightened her grip. He bellowed like a cow in labor. Once again he was made a laughing stock of the community.

Shooting Duck "Brandsdrift"

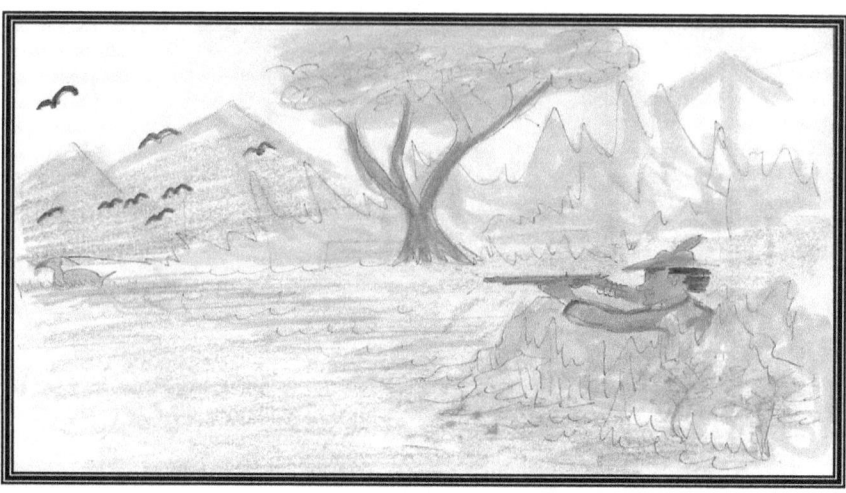

On a certain Sunday I went hunting for duck in between the different farm dams. Not having my favorite shot-gun with, an air gun. The report of the bigger gun would bring the farmers running. On arriving at the dam I saw a nice fat duck wallowing in the water, creeping up silently on hands and knees over the muddy dam wall. Peering over I saw my meal paddling along. I took aim and fired. A "plop" sound was heard. The duck did not move, but carried on swimming. I fired again. No effect. I fired again. No effect. I can't remember how many times I aimed and fired into the ducks posterior, but he had iron as skin. When all my pellets were finished, he suddenly disappeared under the water as a result of all the weight caused by the lead in his body. Diving into the brown murky waters I searched for the duck in the dam floor. Eventually I got hold of a foot. With a gasp I heaved myself above the water level, the duck on tow. Being late for dinner I quickly threw it over my shoulder and trotted homewards. On arriving home with the soggy dead bird it was quickly defeathered. The whole family was waiting mouth watering expectantly for the promised meal. We all could smell the delicious smell of the meal, with local herbs, salt and spices cooking in the three legged iron pot. When the feast arrived, it turned into a disaster. In between the sweet meat we had mouthfuls of air gun lead. Spitting these out, my family was not amused at all. The angry farmer came to my Dad at the store, inquiring after his prize duck, now missing. My Dad feinted surprised knowing nothing. My air-gun was confiscated for the next month.

My earliest memories were of that great mystic granite mountain called Thaba Nchu. We used to love and enjoy climbing and taking races to the top. Climbing meant liking at your footing in case of slipping and sliding down which could mean loosing the race. [Aussie was usually the winner having a heart beat of less that 40. At high school he received his Northern Natal colours in the mile. My youngest brother Mike would excel even more by receiving colours in the Transvaal province. He also received, the envied, 15 time green badge for the comrade marathon.] A sudden slip and yell meant a helping hand. Buck, fleet and fast of foot were common and numerous … a great joy to look at their graceful movement, speed and power sure footing from rock to rock never loosing their balance or failing down a precipice. Dassies or rock rabbits were staring at us secretly, as most of the time they were hidden between rock crevices or bushes. Their favorite past time was lying under the sun having a permanent siesta. At the top looking down thought of wonder and excitement would enter my mind. At a height of 1000ft standing in the thin, cool, fresh air, the eyes searching the horizon. In the hazy distance you could see the city of Bloemfontein, in the opposite direction of the Maluties. In the winter they stood majestically white capped. The wind from them meant a reminder of the cold to come.

At the base of the mountain to this day standing the two houses next to each other, the one thatch the other with a zinc roof. A dam stood above them feeding the cattle. They happily drank thirstily from the murky brownish water. Horizontally along the dam wall stood rows of bushes and trees, as if to guard the wall. Below this is an orchard and veggie garden, watered daily by means of rows of irrigation channels. Leading to the twin farm houses a winding dirt road with intervals of 20m were small water breakers to deflect rain when it rained hard. The main road to Bloemfontein and Durban ran at right angles to this road. The entrance gate advertised "Merino Sheep for Sale" looking at the donga running in front of the gate with a small bridge, reminded me of an amusing incident. My mother had just got her driving license, but did not have must practice. My Dad played golf that afternoon in Tweespruit, gave quick last minute instructions of how to slow down and apply the foot brake. Unfortunately on arrival at the Glamorgan gate at high speed, we ploughed diagonally into the muddy "sloot". Six Afikaner oxen had to pull the once maroon 1950 Ford out after a great heave and a crack of resounding whip lash. My mother refused to drive again, her nerves shattered. As mentioned before, Brands drift was where we as Girds lived. The Brand drift of today looks very depressing comparing to 50 years ago. The homestead is a pile of stones, the many trees now far and between scraggly lots. The whole area looks morbid, a memory of the good days gone by.

Cloud burst

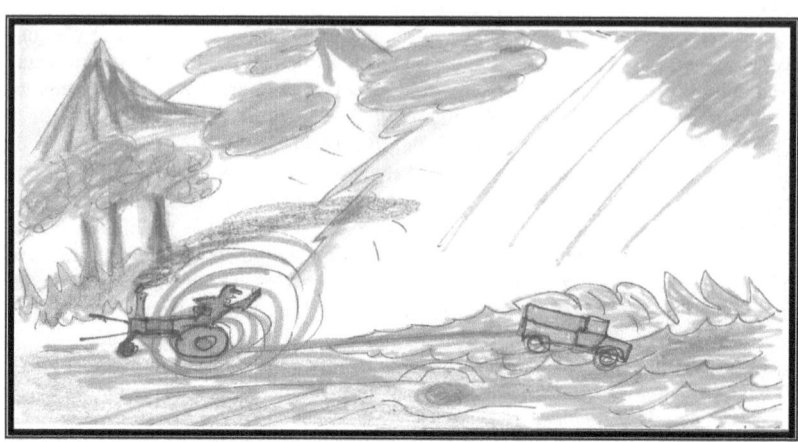

It was the year 1950 a hot and windless day. My Dad had just bought a second had Ford V8 green coloured, with a canopy made of taught canvas. As the custom was most of the farmers in the area of Tweepruit had just played golf. We were all in a good mood as my Dad had just won a prize, a lucky hole in one on the notorious 17th hole.

The golf course had ringed about it a great number of huge eucalyptus trees, the fragrant aroma, overpowering. Today they look like a scraggly lot, over the years the worse for wear. In the winter months their huge ranches could barely hold the white caked snow. The cracking and straining you could hear, when looking for a lost golf ball. Luckily the local Basotho were wrapped in their thick multicolored blankets, the chilling icy "Maluti" berg wind trying to get in.

To come back to my trust life story, we all went to the local drinking hole, Tweespruits hotel, their parents were relaxing and enjoying drinks and playing snooker, black ball wins. Us children, my two brothers, our cousins Ann, Joy and the Orchison's and many more were playing hide and seek in the shadows of the buildings. After 12 many jokes and farmer tales only they could understand, we left for home. The roar of the starting cars could be heard, their unsteady head lights yellowy etched against the gloomy tree foliages, in the night. The Gird family now behind the new 1952 Ford of the Higgs's rich in our eyes on the way to there farm Glaorgan, the home stead nestling against the mighty crags of Thaba Chu.

Early the following morning after a hearty "farmers" break fast the same as today we were ready to leave for our home Brandsdrift lying between the town of Exselsior and the English name, Westminister. On the way to the bakkie, all eyes as the custom is to look at the sky for signs of welcome rain. The clouds were building up ominously in the south. The wind starting to blow harder, foreboding were those mean looking Cumulus, a menace in the distance, my mother feeling apprehensive quickly had us loaded to be on our way. Down the sloping narrow farm road we drove towards the main dirt road. It started raining softly, then with more meaning, the wind screen wipers in motion, and the road ahead dimly seen through the pouring rain. At the top of the steep gradient moving over the hill, the gravel road now a quagmire of mud, we came to a slithering stand still. The radiator was now pouring hot steam. Our situation a predicament, we were in big trouble. To make matters worse we ere stuck in a sloot where the churning brown mountain water came rushing on to us. Water was slamming us side ways. We were huddled together frightened, Mom saying the Hail-Mary softly. We started to float.

Unknown to us my dad had already ran for help, the nearest farm a mile away. He was my hero a mighty soldier having shot many of the enemy. His flashing smile always there. The bakkie was now on its side ready to tip over. The roar of the cutting rain bearing winds now a howl, the lightning blinding the thunder like a great lion in pain, "hang on, I have come with help" a muffled cry was heard through the dim rushing water. It was pitching dark. A sudden jerk was felt, it was the end, and farmer's hands had tied a thick manila rope to the back bumper. On the other end of the taught rope was a Massy-Fergeson tractor. We were on the way to safety. Our own muffle cries not heard, us huddled together hope was dimly near. The tractor's wheels were spinning madly, the mud flung rotating in the rainy air, its driver grimly determined the bystanders now many, ready to assist. As the tractor pulled and moving; our own predicament was far from over, danger close by. As we moved, so did the raging, gushing stream cover the V-8 and us at the back? We were like a U-boat to be stranded on the beach. The strong rope doing its job, it did not break. Emerging out of the dark morass of eminent drowning, the bystanders thought, they saw a muddy mole emerging out of those swirling waters, danger averted. A family now safe, mothers sigh of relief. Strong arms hoisted us to warmth and safety. A hot delicious mug of coffee trusted into our hands, "Are you ok!" We were asked, every one happy it was over.

Years later when ever I pass that place past the sloot, I remember everything vividly, and how Mom spoke of the day we were saved by prayers. The cloud burst its sounds a dim memory, not forgotten.

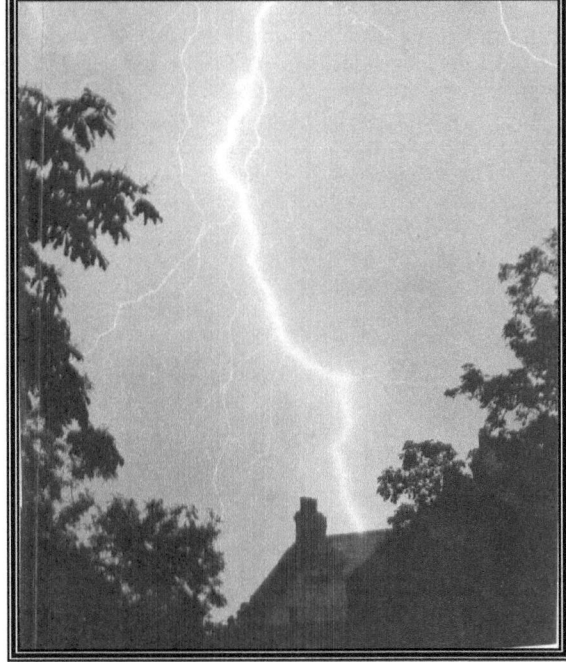

Mike an awkward moment

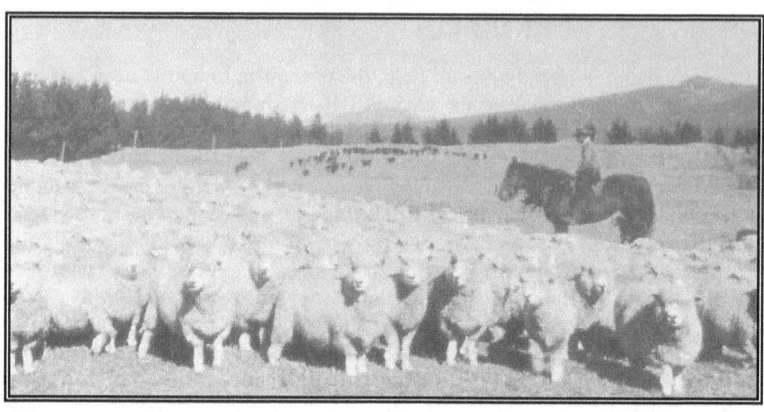

Mike my youngest brother took three years to start talking. We thought he may have been slow, but he was to prove us all wrong, showing a quick and agile brain for facts and figures. His three degree would prove it. At that time we were young teenagers. On the farm it was lambing time again, their bleating could be heard for miles around, their echoes rebounding from the cliff faces far above the farm across the mountains. Being a warm day we both wore shorts, a mitigating factor. Mike and I were up early to enjoy the lambs being fed either by hand or via the mother sheep. The black farm hands knew their job and the lambs were eager to drink the satisfying cow's milk from bottles. A lot o them had milk and wanted more, they followed Mike and me as we made a quick retreat, climbing through the barbed wire fence. Three lambs chased after us, I escaped unscathed, but Mike was not so lucky. As he climbed through, his one leg on the other side, the other following, a lamb darted towards his private parts and hung on. Obviously it thought is his mother's teat. Mike turned a beetroot red with embarrassment. The show was over quicker than it started. The lamb retreated not satisfied that it was not the real thing. Mike and I were too shy to talk about it to this day. Mike take this story as a joke!

Aussie the giver

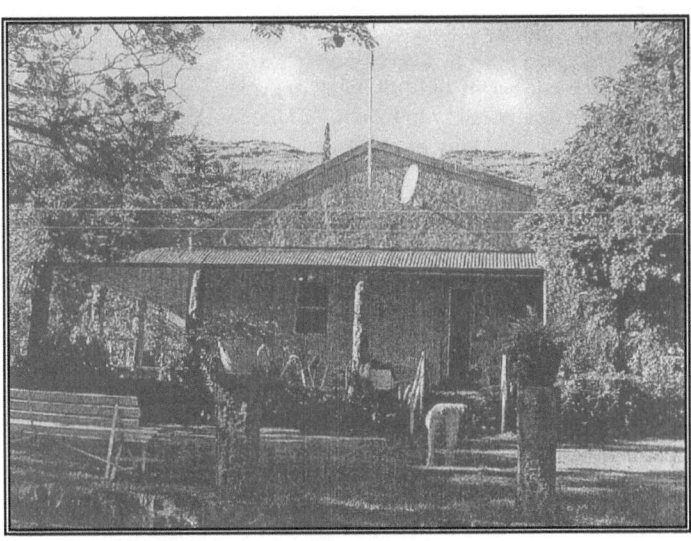

Aussie was a very loving and giving person. What he gave to whom and when did not concern him. On this occasion the circumstances fitted like a surgeon's glove, the timing of the giving hilarious. On the Glamorgan farm the fun stated. The English are sticklers for tradition and protocol. 10 o'clock was always tea time. The best china cups were brought out by the servant girl, there being his ranking visitors, my brother Aussie. My Uncle was in a serious mood, while the holistic ritual of pouring the tea was being done, the old garden boy was busy pruning the roses, below the verandah where they sat chatted. On impulse Buffy got up, excused himself to go to the toilet, Aussie sitting, waiting for his big farmer uncle. He caught sight of the garden boy perspiring in the red hot sun. Feeling sorry for the old man, jumped up with the beautiful hand made tea cup with gold ring rim, gave it to the black man to drink from. Standing next to him offering him tea, took the gardener totally by surprise. Not being used to the white "morena" offering him anything, much less tea from his own tea cup. He stood paralyzed, rooted on the spot. At that critical moment in time Buffy arrived. He could not believe what he was seeing. He let out a lion's roar. "Aussie what are you doing?" The gardener carried on pruning. It was needless to say the high atmosphere of comradeship came to a sudden end the tea on the verandah went cold. Aussie's giving was not appreciated that day.

Primary School

Unfortunately my first years at Primary School at Westminister can be remembered when on the second day of school I was given a lift by avery smelly "taxi driver" whose sweat dripped on to my back. I sat across the cross bar of the "dik wiel" bicycle as the taxi driver peddle up the winding bumpy gravel road 10 miles away to school. The school was a one building, one room, verandah in front, with steps leading to the front gate, and a main road across leading to and from Bloemfontein and Durban. On the opposite side was the single railway track, the station being Westminster. Steam locomotion chugged its way past the school daily, causing us all to cough. Today the only sign of a school are a few stones and bushes. Memories there of bring back a chocking feeling in my throat. Feelings of nostalia, a past happy remembered. Concerning the passenger train there was a story about British troops who fought during the 2nd Boer War. They thought prickly pears, growing along the railway tracks, were real pears, picking them from the couch windows. Not knowing how to peal them, they tried to remove the prickles without success, some put them hands full into their pockets or vests. To their horror rashes occurred, pain and army Doctors had to remove the prickles. Locals told them to use butter or fat to remove the prickly pear prickles. Some said it was a silly "attack" by the boers, or blacks who told them how delicious they eat to eat when ripe.

In std. 2 our whole school of 20 went on a trip through that town to visit the last resting place of the great Basotho mountain king Moshweshwe. Pictures always show him sitting in thought with his conical light straw hat on a ling stemmed pipe in his left gnarled black hand. Sad eyes fading in old age. As a young man he was a dynamic leader, organizer against the Boers. When danger of invasion threatened he and his tribe would quickly under covered nights, escape to a huge mountain called Thaba Bosiu "mountain of the night". Here was only one way to go up, a narrow path. No one not even the mighty Boers could overcome them, once entrenched. Louw Wepener a brave soldier tried to crawl up through the path but was met with a savage hale of stones. His comrades had to very carefully fetch his broken body when the moon faded behind a cloud. He was named posthumously a hero, by the Boers. A siege of that annexable mountain was fruitless; they gave up and went home, a victory for the mountain dwellers with stolen cattle joyously stayed safely on their mountain of the night.

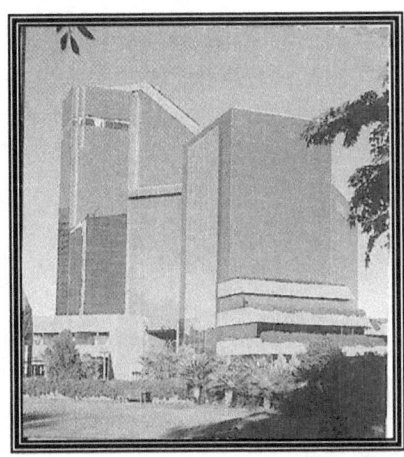

Westminister not having std. 3 forced me to go to CBC, Bloemfontein, where I boarded with a family for a 'long' year. I really enjoyed "big School" playing soccer, athletics and cricket. As a catholic I went for my first communion, confession and later conformation. To send you on your way the Bishop would give a gentle slap across the face! The happiest days were those when holidays arrived. The adventure would begin on the passenger train. This steam driven locomotion would belch very dark smoke and to look out the carriage window would mean stinging soot in your eyes. The clicked-clack is still ringing in my ears. Usually the train was the milk train or "melk trein" stopping at every siding to drop off or on loading milk. The black passengers were behind the loco, a packed mass of jolly talking without restraint echo. The "whites" in a few carriages behind seated in subdued silence. As the train made its way winding along the green land, the locos shrill high pitched voice would warn of an approaching depot. The many black and white patched mild cows were a witness to the farming milk trade. The friendly conductor would share his "pad kos" with me having been prepared by the "tannie" on approaching Westminister would call me to get off, or land up in the Lesotho capital Masuru.

Northern Natal

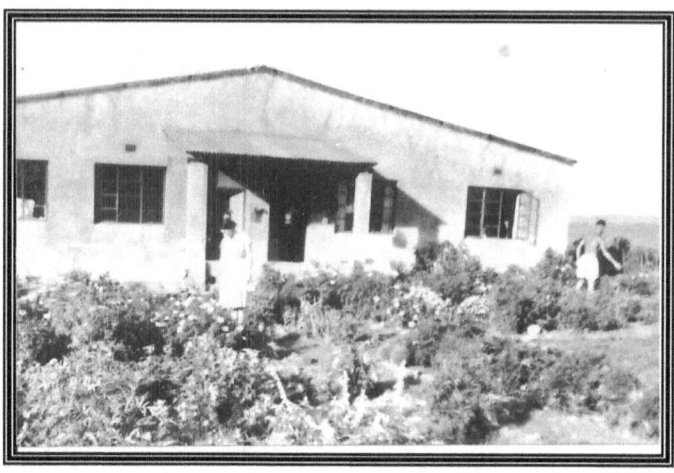

My Dad rented a trading store at a place called Oulaar, 20 km from Newcastle, which for us, as a family would prove to be disastrous financially. In std. 4 would be the last year at Brands drift and then off to Northern Natal. Oulaar Mountain was my favorite haunt to look for and find old bones. In those days the dinky toys had just come out and us young boys had a passion for collecting them. To add to my low budget pocket money, I had to make plan to add to the little I had stored away for those were poor days.

The best way then was to collect old bones, these my dad sold in bulk to a passing agent who in turn sold them to a factory that made strong glue for all purposes, especially for leather and upholstery. To get bones had to take a bit of organization. A few black friends and a mule were hired. Along with 10 empty maze meal bags, off we went to the small mountain called "Oulaar". As we traveled towards it through the veld and path ways we would start looking around for bones. When we found them the bags had to be filled. I always had my air-gun with me. It was easy to handle but quite heavy. On the top was a small hole with a small moving door with handle to open and close to allow the pellets in. I shot many ringkal snakes, doves, mearcats and rabbits for food for the black gang to eat. Once on the mountain we would find more than enough old bones. This was hard work, we had to climb and scratch around looking for bones along the steep cliff edges, it would take the whole day to get there and back, tied.
The next day would be to sort out the different size bones, weighed, counted and the big moment the pay out. The mule had to be fed, the black gang paid and of cause the money counted to buy the dinky toys at Oulaar trading store. When my dad went to town I would obviously go with to by my well earned dinky toy.

We eventually moved to town, where my Mom got a job as the secretary to our School Newcastle High. My Dad became the manager of the local milk depot. We became socially more active, the Dowlings being our best friends and via the church as altar boys. The priest friendly and outgoing, the convent sister, made me think of a vocation as a priest. My Dad was very happy to hear the news as being a Irish, a priest in the family would mean a blessing. The Bishop interviewed me and in the year 1961 I started at the Catholic Seminary in Boksburg.

Foxy

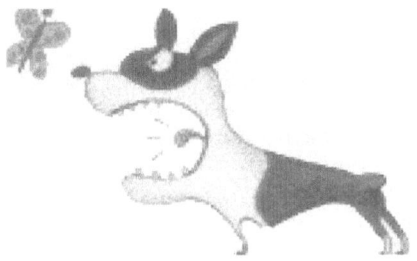

Northern Natal 1959

Foxy had one eye and three legs, a fox terrier with white and black patches. He belonged exclusively to Austin my one brother. This funny looking dog helped him to retrieve what he shot. He was also the best shot; my mother said it was because of his bright blue eyes. I on the other hand was a poor shooter, explaining why I always missed that "Berg-duif" even at close range. Only at the age of 14, did the Oculist in Newcastle pronounce that I was very short sighted and should wear glasses until the age of 50 and then it won't be necessary. I have since passed that age ten years ago and still wear them.

On a certain morning as the sun was rising in the east, us three brothers were on the go, hunting for those elusive "berg-doves, we fanned out in a line, rifles at the ready lying in the shoulder, as soldiers did. We approached a 90° cliff face. This was a mountain, looking like a fortress hiding its inhabitants, our prey. The fat birds were sitting high above us as if laughing at us. Realizing that our approach was wrong we started climbing. After an hours steep climbing, we approached them from the side the drop from above was at least 15m, falling would mean your end. The colour of the cliff face was a weather beaten brown-gray, covered with birds and dassie droppings. From out of the side of the cliff, laterally grew branches bushes and shrubs. So in this atmosphere and tension the adrenalin pumping we crawled, stopping, peering in to the gloom for our prey. One foot would step in front of the other carefully, the gun at the ready. Foxy our own Jock of the bush veld was ahead, sniffing, peering in a head, ready to jump into action at a rifles sound. We don't know how he managed to balance himself on that precarious footing, with only three legs and one eye.

The story behind those gruesome injuries is a muddled one. This is what the herdsman told us of how it happened, he being the key witness in this "case". Foxy sniffing the air caught the whiff if a bitch on heat. Unfortunately there was a hound before him. This hound was "on the job". Wanting a piece of the action, Foxy lost control and blindly went on to the attack. Eyeing the hanging Rodweiler's testicles, flying, he sunk his teeth in them. With a terrible howl of pain, and losing his bitch under him, penis dangling, he went after our Foxy, realizing his mess, take our Jock of the bushveld, bounded away for his life. In one direction ran the bitch, after him lose at his heels was "Satan" the wounded Rodweiler, a mask of hatred, his prey close. Being a bigger dog he caught up, his most powerful jaws sinking into Foxy's left upper leg. Foxy was caught as if in a devils clamp, a bloody vice of sharp teeth. Rolling over they went a bundle of fur, rolling in the dust, the blood pouring out. With a might crunch the leg bones crumbled, his leg came off, in "Satan's" mouth. Foxy now on three legs, hobbled away to safety. He was mistaken for a second time, "Satan" now in one of those bloody lusts to go for the kill. His giant jaws closed over the fox terriers head, it was the end! Out of no where a helping hand arrived, by means of a mighty "knop-kierie", our very highly muscled black Zulu herdsman struck the dog. The black antagonist dog, now with a cracked skull retreated dizzly away with a cry and muffled roar.

Wrapping Foxy in a Basotho blanket, now a bloody mess, Jafta was on his pony. He raced to my Dads shop. Dad had to play Veterinarian, for the closest one was too far away. He having some knowledge of first aid stopped the blood and bandaged the dog.   Aussie was in tears. Miraculously this hardy terrier mended fast. Love, cow's milk and close attention did the trick. The horrible and terrifying ordeal was over, but his scares were not. It can be said that in the future Foxy will be more circumspect in approaching a bitch on heat.

Back to our hunting story, I was difficult terrain to hunt in, the footing precarious. One had would be the on the rifle, the other holding onto a protruding brunch of bush. Suddenly out of the gloom screeched out a guinea-fowl in flight. Two shots went off, two simultaneous thuds of bullets finding their mark heard. Two whoops of delight! I, coming out of one side of the bush and Aussie out of the other both claming the kill. We descended on the lifeless bird, I had shot first, no he shot first, we argued. Mike now a bystander could no take sides; he had heard one shot, some one cleverer took over. Foxy! Like a flash of greased lighting, his jaws firmly gripping the fowl, off he ran homewards, we were after him, shouting.   My mother had anticipated food on the way and had organized three legged pot, already steaming over a open air fire of dry wood.

Forgotten was the argument, the present mattered. The meat mixed with fresh veggies was most delicious, today we would call it "potjie-kos" others would describe it as finger-licking-good, with a happy tune of "it's nice, it's nice"

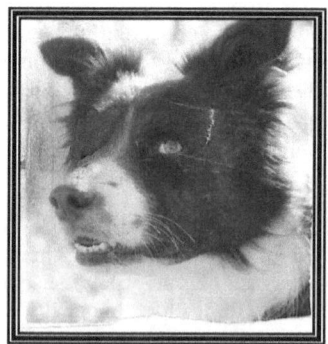

Sick of Pumpkin

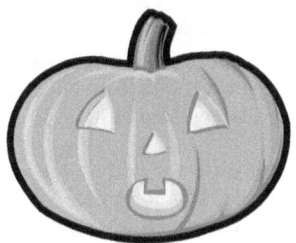

Newcastle Northern Natal 1960

As a family we enjoyed both the town life and farm life. Fresh milk we could get at the dairy where my Dad worked as a manger for a rich farmer. Our house was built adjacent to the depot. The main Durban road to Johannesburg ran next to our front door. In the near distance you could hear the rail way trucks and carriages being shunted, the great steam locomotive blowing and pushing them to their sidings. The tall chimneys of the massive steel works could be seen, belching smoke and unhealthy smog. As you came into town you went over a concrete bridge, under which ran from North to South a clear stream of icy berg water. What spoiled the fresh air from those mountains was the steel works smog, black and unsightly in the early morning.

Newcastle was good to us, after our disastrous stay at Oulaar 20 miles outside of town. Our financial went from bad to worse. "Five pounds a month" my mother said. The area was where the poorest of the poor lived, so as a business we could not survive. To go to school we had to walk the five miles to a huge gate, belonging to a rich farmer who hired white maid and flew a two winged biplane. His wife was a teacher in Newcastle, who took us to and from school daily. Being always late, she kept the 1960 Ford V8 at a 120 mph speed. The car used to shake and strain to get there, but safely we did!

An unfortunate accident happened to my brother Mike being only 10 years old. Coming down at speed with his "dik wiel" bike, he got into trouble at a sloot and corrugation in this un-kept dirt road. Falling with the bike on top of him he let out a terrible scream of pain, the lower leg broken, the tibia bone splintered, the blood pouring into his shoe and made a furrow on the bloody gravel.

I stood petrified, from shock and not knowing how to help or stop the blood flow. Having first aid training now, I can only look back in retrospect. I started running to the nearest farm house, the home stead of the Du Toits. On hearing about the accident he started to International V8 and came roaring down the twin track road, through the open rickety gate to where Mike as lying. He quickly put a make-shift tourniquet on. Once the blood had stopped and a piece of plank tied to the leg to keep it straight, we make for my Dad's work. Shocked parents they put him gently into the maroon Ford, the blood having stopped, but no end to his sobbing. It took him two weeks to recover, but his lower leg would never be straight again. Being still not well he started demanding that he get the same good as that he was used to while he was in the hospital. Fried bacon, poached eggs not too soft, three pieces of toast with butter and not our cheap margarine we used. His antics caused all of us to laugh, as it wasn't often some one gave my Dad a lot of 'back-chat'. My Dad was not amused.

Being in town gave us a piece of both worlds, the out door and town life. We would go visiting our pals on their farms or plots, there we would be either shooting with the double barreled shot gun, our favourite because you couldn't miss. Boating, hiking in the bush and having a good time as young teenagers would do. The black people here were far different to the Basotho I was used to. First I would have to learn their difficult Zulu clicking sounding language, the opposite to Southern Sotho of which language I knew from birth.

They were a taller race, blacker with different body odor, more pungent. Once aroused and angry he would done his fighting regalia, a "knop kierie" in hand and the famous Charka Zulu oval cow hide shield. With blood thirsty cries, rattles and whistles blowing the tribe would be on the move, as if to war. One such a black, a farmers shepherd a deaf-mute, lived in a normal Zulu conical straw hut, he had the mentioned problem, but his other problem was worse. He lived on his own for a reason, his penis was too big. If it did not hang down between his legs, he would be raping one of his sheep. The Zulu women were terrified of his advances, he becoming a recluse. Of course the farmer got to hear by means of the "grape vine". On examining the said sheep, the Vet had to give surgery to the vagina as if some and the anuses of others. After a beating at the local SAP, 20 lashes with a cane, he was castrated by the local doctor.

One a certain weekend which I will not forget Richard Tourle, Aussie and I hopped on our bikes, loaded to go camping in the berg. On reaching a suitable camping site next to a broad brown river, we bedded down for the night. We went hungry because I being too hungry ate up all the biltong and carrots. They were not impressed with me at all. During the night a storm unexpectedly broke loose, over our heads. In desperation we headed to the nearest farm a dim light in the distance gloom. On arriving there we were welcome with open arms, our mud washed off in a steaming hot tub, and clothed warmly. At 2 am we had a big porridge plate of yellow pumpkin. On this was put a blob of farmers home made butter, and a dash of sugar. Round about 6 the morning the menu was repeated, this time with milk. At noon it was pumpkin again, in its peal, having been baked in the oven. This went on for three days, pumpkin coming out of our ears! On Sunday, after prayers we were treated to fried fritters and there local jam, made of a type of watermelon, it was delicious.

Obviously they were very poor. It was the first time I had seen a pig on a diet; its ribs were sticking out. Their old horse was a white colour but now a sickly gray, with a hobble. They had no tractor, the four brown tawny Afrikaner oxen were in spanned to do the ploughing, and the drivers cracking the bull hide whip heard echoing among the mountain cliffs. Monday being a public holiday we had to say our goodbyes, with sighs of relief. Walking to the said river we fetched our transport, back home we pedaled with a pumpkin under the arm for mother and father to enjoy.
Having had a "pumpkin" of a weekend!

When ever Martie, my wife, makes pumpkin fritters, I refuse to eat it.
I wonder why?

Cross-country running - 1960

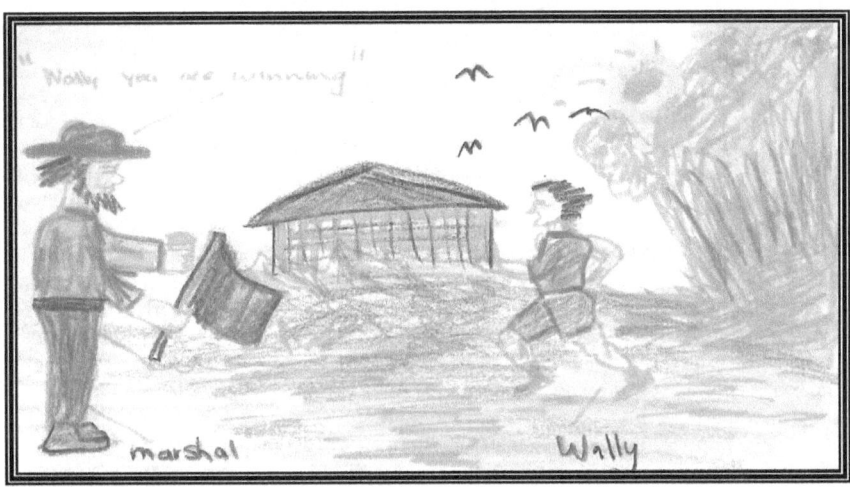

Newcastle Northern Natal

I would like to tell you about my cross –country running experience. I was in Standard 7 at the time. Included in the school program was athletics. I was very good at the 100m, 200m, 400m,and 800m but not further, I was then out of breath. My brother Austin on the other hand had a heart beat of 40, making him a better candidate for the longer distances. He was also the current cross- country champion for the under 14 team in the Northern Natal.

On that afternoon plus-minus 400 boys and girls gathered together for the annual New Castle High cross-country race. We all stood crouching in readiness for the starter's gun to signal the take-off. Not being very interested in the proceedings I stood idly at the back of the "ready" pack, with a start I heard the crack of the gun, in a matter of minutes everyone was out of sight. Non-pulsed I stood alone "Why are they running so fast? I thought. Off I went in hot pursuit. At about a mile further on I got lost, "which way to turn, left or right? No marshals were in sight. I turned to the left, trotting in those days would be called a "Zulu trot" a steady slow jog.

Unexpectedly in front of me loomed a thickly foliaged clump of trees, wattle and dense bush. This small forest it was dark and gloomy, it was also difficult to weave my way, ducking and diving to avoid being scratched, the thorns sharp. The running slowed to a walk, the higher branches had cut off the suns rays. The under growth had a sharp pungent odor, a low life of its own. On some places I had to crawl, wiggle and frog leg to get through the thorns and under lying branches impeding the way. The dark gave slowly away to stronger light, I was through!

Stumbling into the open and sunlight, I had to rub my eyes to focus properly to see in which way was the direction of the school, and hostel, near to it. Coming to a unexpected road crossing, I met a marshal, with his flag and juice. Nearly colliding into each other, me coming from the wrong direction, he said "Wally you are doing very well, you are coming first". Spurred on by this unexpected good news, changing gear gleefully from a slow trot to a fast run, the end line being my objective, a record to be broken! The perspiration now pouring off me I approached the school grounds. Those who saw me started cheering and clapping hands. "Come on Wally, you are winning", I was now at full speed to receive my due honors. Looking behind me I saw no one in pursuit. Suddenly it struck me, I had inadvertently taken a short-cut and if I did come first it would have been a default, and not only illegal but a big lie.

The crowds ere cheering madly, they had a unexpected new champion. Why was Wally running so fast today? Now in a quandary, eyeing a ablution block to the left, I feinted a sudden limp and made for the toilets. Luckily for me this was situated on a bend in between a lot of trees. No one was there at that spot, it suited me, at speed I ducked into the smelly building, went into a booth and sat down to wait for the ones who had run the race legally to pass by, it wasn't long when before the crowd started cheering and clapping. A hour went by, when I emerged shame facedly, limping just in time to see my brother Austin receiving the "honors", no one up to this day asked me what happened or why I didn't finish, or where was my "national record!"

My mother did ask me where I got so many cuts and bruises, but my clever answer was from a recent cowboy film starring John Wayne, where he would always say "it goes with the badge". I gave the same answer!

I lost a close friend

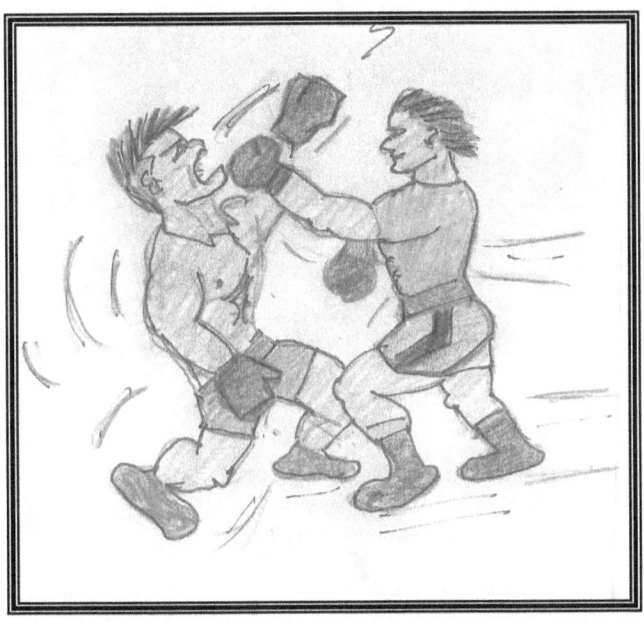

It was holiday time and we were one our way to Newcastle, Natal in a train. We traveled from the Transvaal over the great winding Drakensburg range. The shrill call of the locomotive, its churning grinding wheels a thrill to hear. My friend John was much exited to come with me on the journey. It would be his first over night and a new experience for him, not having left Johannesburg before. My whole family welcomed us with open arms at the station. To make my friend enjoy himself more we treated him to the out door life, shooting ducks, sailing, bicycling. We were active boys. On a certain day he looked quiet moody and wanted to do some boxing as he claimed to be a champion at his club. We donned the boxing gloves; Mike my youngest brother faced him for a friendly demonstration of his reputed skills. The bout took place in the garage. With out warning he put down Mike with a combination of punches, Mike now terrified let out a scream. I quickly intervened, Mike off to mother to stop a bleeding nose. I had to revenge this unfair and bloody assault. Donning the gloves I was in a fury. Facing my opponent I challenged him to do the same to me. Surprised was written on his face "You are my Friend" he mumbled. "I don't want to hurt you." With all my strength and power I attacked him.

The first punch caught him on the curled lips, the second on the right aggressive eye. He staggered back in a daze, ducking and weaving in the classical boxing style. The swollen lips were now puffed up, his eye closing, aching and paining. His head was pounding and throbbing. To my surprise he ran out of the garage with a might. Yell of frustration. Throwing the gloves off, went to my mother. He as a guest had been treated badly and wanted to go home now! My mother said he was booked on the next train home. I had lost a friend.

Brown River rafting 1960

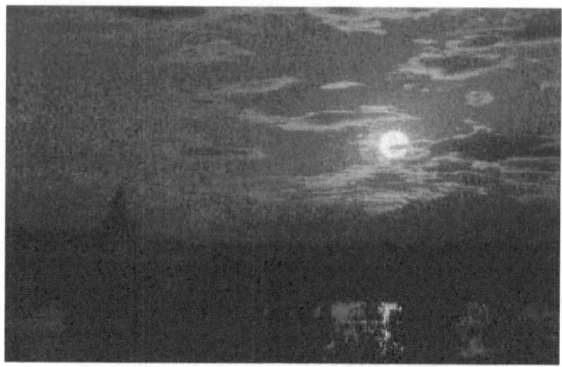

A slow meandering Buffels river made its way in snaky curves past the sleepy town. I t was deep but not very wide. A long its banks grew indifferent shapes and sizes of Weeping Willows and further out the Natal Black wattle, dense and hard to cut. The river water was filthy, and full of the dreaded Balazia, a small weevil if it got up your privates in to the bladder would cause that grave sickness. It was more prevalent among the blacks.

Straddled across this water course, was at its narrowest part, a rickety wooden bridge, swinging dangerously as you walked slowly carefully across to the other side. Inadvertly falling in would mean food for the waiting Piranhas, and the wicked teeth of the hungry crocodiles.

A good friend of mine Hansie Venter, and the rest of the gang, liked to go river brown-river rafting as apposed to white-river rafting, obviously because of the dirty brown colour of the stagnant water, stinking to high heavens. The "boats" were made up of 44 gallon drums, fastened tightly together by means of manilla rope. On top of these drums was tied the wooden platform nailed together. Weekends we would push these from the bushes where they were hidden and the pulled into the waiting river. Usually there were three floats and 10 boys. Once in the river it would be a matter of peddling and paddling hard down river to where we had our hidden camp where we usually spent the night.

On that steamy hot day we headed paddling as per usual to the camp. We divided the chores between us; one would go hunting with the "22" rifle, a sharp report of the shot could be hear, not long after the hunter would appear with his trophy, a large long legged hare. A hole in the head, the pros would quickly strip the corpse of its soft leather skin, and intestines, these would be buried. The leather kept to be hung up to dry in the wind and sun, sold later for some pocket money. The dry wood fire was in full swing, the black three legged pot steaming. Into the pot we put the rabbit now cut up, with different types of local veggies and salt.

One of the kids had a mouth organ, the rest of us sang, the words unknown. With full belly we all crept in to our sleeping bags, tired from all the paddling, we were all fast asleep, only the cold moon and stars were our witness. A gentle snoring could be heard.

Far to the west a storm was growing, in that cold night. To the south stood the great heights of mountain steeples, capped with a touch of snow, it wasn't winter yet. A draught of hot air met head on with the higher cold strata. This friction caused a dramatic change in the atmosphere, Cumulus gathered. Thunder erupted. Jagged frightening lightning appeared. Hail and rain poured from the heavens. A full blooded storm was in full swing, the cliffs, dongas, slots and rivulets were now filling up at an alarming rate and over flowing quickly. The stark outlines of the jagged black cliffs were highlighted when the heavens lit up. The rolling thunder followed, a crashing echo among the great rocks of this Darkensburgs mountain range was heard. The water now flowing up to twenty times its volume was ready to break the banks of all rivers in is way. The unsuspecting campers, far to its east knew nothing of this looming, threatening dangerous course of nature.

As fate had its way they were directly in the path of the monstrous flood, on its way. This was all happening in the depth of the night, while nature was busy with its secrets of heavenly motions.

When morning came we boys, the campers were busy having our last cup of steaming coffee, ready to paddle back home and to church as it was a Sunday. The clouds were gathering but were not intent on that, but on the return journey the heavy paddling upstream – a mile away, to be where we would pull the rafts out of the water, hide them and troop back home to a welcome bath.

Unknown to us an unwelcome bath was waiting for us in the shape of the storm raging towards us. A tidal wave of about 2m was approaching at high speed, flattening all in its path. In its wake were broken dam walls, flooded framers crops, those who built mud huts on the river banks, or sheep and oxen gone with the flow of destruction. We were on our way, the water level started climbing higher and higher, an effort to paddle, we were not going backwards nor forward. The water now a boil, a roar of sound, our frantic cries for naught, the wind now a howl, the once elegant willow trees were now bent over and backwards to breaking point, cracking. The great tidal wave struck, we submerged like sinking submarines. The cascade pouring over us, now separated from our boats we could only struggle to get to the safety of the river edge, now a quagmire of mud and broken branches. Here we held on for dear life, water pressure on the hands and arms to force away too awesome, we were going to be swept away.

Just as suddenly as it happened, just as suddenly the water flow pulling us to our doom, it stopped, the tidal wave had past, the storm had abated. We were safe, our drums were gone but we were alive, a sorry sight for sore eyes, our troop of boys made their way home, bedraggled.

We eventually did get our hot bath, but our parents were not aware of the terrible danger their children had gone through, nor did my parents know what really happened to me, when Brown River rafting became a danger for life.

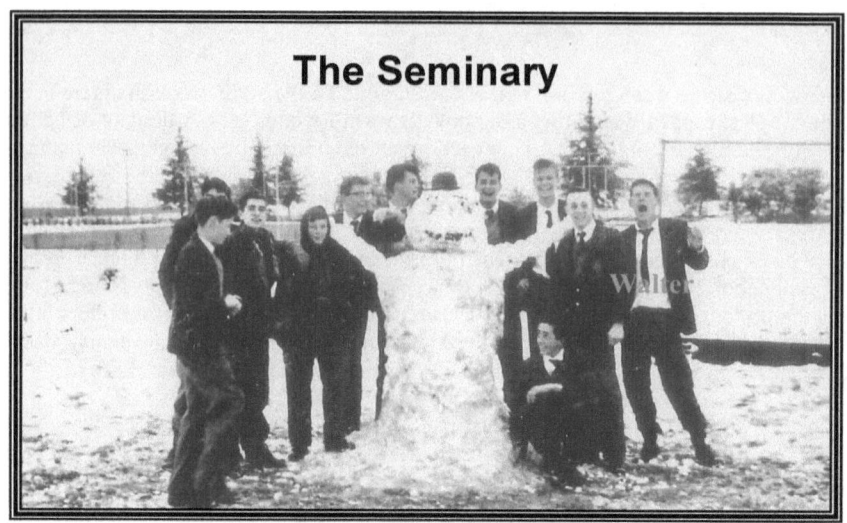

The Seminary

Walter and Seminarians in the Snow in 1962

I still remembered arriving at the seminary, the spiraling tower to the one side, were the chapel was two Franciscans priests brown robed, rope around the waist cross hanging in front, welcome me and other candidate priests. The massive building was built in the shape of a large L. The top stories were the living quarters for us and the brown robed teachers of the church. To describe them was not difficult. The senior priest white faced, a hair line lip, effeminate, the hands of a piano player, a musician, and the big boss in charge. The other an Fr Stan an ex sports man in weight lifting. He was a very strong and friendly man to look up too. He was invaluable to me in my studies especially Latin, the language of the church then. The rules of standard of conduct was very high and sever, it would be my army training which I missed. Both priests were from the land of the Shamrock, their home far away. The Green Ireland, their accent strange sounding to me with my background Free State Farming. My languages were African in nature, Sotho, Zulu, coming recently from Natal, Afrikaans and accented English. Their "sing song" sounds. We all got used to the rules which were simple: no talking when there was retreat, no talking after lights out at 10 pm!

With out me knowing I would be in a restricted enclosure, and would later be very unhappy, a life not for me, the opposite of my exiting open air life that I was used too. We were led to our dormitories each pupil had a room to himself. In the small room was a bed, cross on the wall, wardrobe and study table. The ablutions were at the end of the dormitory. The two priests in charge had their own quarters. We were awakened by the words "Ave Maria" the answer would be two "Gratia Plenna" which means Hail Mary Full of grace. The blurry eyed masturbators would line up for confession the next morning. Those who could not control this habit would have to leave"master the bodies' desirers" was the pass word or go.

The mornings started at 5 o'clock, you got up immediately, mass, prayers, study and breakfast, then off to Christian Brothers College by bike. I got on very well with the brothers they were very friendly and helpful. Their dedication amazed me, their spirit cheerful. This motivated me to study harder. At the seminary it was a case of who was the holiest to make an impression on the priest in charge. We were drilled in the art of singing, public speaking, plays and prayer. We were being prepared for the future as priest of the Holy Roman Catholic Church to fight evil. The world outside had to be conquered for Christ. As priest we were to make three vows.

1. Chastity (no sex, or marriage)
2. Poverty (you don't own anything all belongs to the church)
3. Obedience (which means going any where in the world when ordered by the Bishop). Strict discipline was the order of the day.

 Total silence was allowed with no talking. Weekends would be spent listening to priest from the major seminary to exhort us on. I enjoyed sport, as too much of something made me morbid. At CBC I played for the first team rugby, playing at Ellis Park in the finals.

The austere and strict seminary also had it funny and amusing incidents. My first and formal dinner was a total disaster. The dinning room tables and chairs ere in a U shaped configuration. At the top end of the U sat two priest and the proctors. At the tables facing each other the candidates were seated. At the open end of the U was the lectern from where the readings were done. From the time you walked in, you were observed by all. No one told me. I was quiet hungry that day and could not wait to eat. Directly after the readings I sat down. The waiting bread went quickly into the soup with a plonk, due to the sudden silence the sound was heard by all. Blowing hard through the steamy broth I heard a sharp high pitched reprimand. "Walter, stand up please! Open mouthed, some giggling while the dumb founded students stared at me. Slowly I stood up shamed faced, the worst moment of my life, being the center of attention and being made a fool of. "At least the farmer made life more interesting" was said in the corridors. Obviously I got the lecture on good manners and dinner protocol.

I managed to escape initiation; I don't know why the world over effeminate boys and men attract attention. Such was one of the candidates to be initiated that day. Also being new and to be 'run in' he was targeted first. Unluckily for him it rained heavily that morning. The surrounding area was wet. A muddy pool near by was half full, towards this the happy crowd, holding a Lilly white boy on high, a wriggling screaming hysterical priest to be, head long he went flying into the filthy water. With a shriek he, with a mighty and resounding splash. On hauling him out, he looked like a bedraggled meowing cat, muddy and scraggly. Under the icy, cold shower he was cleaned from head to toe. The priests were out for a meeting with the Bishops, the timing just right. The angry effeminate rushed off to the phone to his well-to-do parents. They were not amused at all. Irritated they asked the Father what type of seminary he was running. From that day on no more initiations were done, needless to say our friend did not last long. After much teasing and booing he left for greener fields at the end of that year.

As the long term wore on, we all got irritated and frustrated. Arguments erupted over the smallest difference of opinions. Illegal fights broke out between us; we went to our P.T. officer, who agreed that due to stress boxing gloves were to be used as a form of therapy. Under his guidance and leadership we had bouts of sparring lessons, those who had gripes, boxed first. The swinging arms and fists exploded into action, the spectators roared their approval, each one backing their favorite champion. Bloody noses and puffy eyes were the results, frustrations now a pain in the head. I had my chance at the head prefect, a long and tall fellow. He had an Elvis Presley hair style, a long curl hanging in between his devil eyes, long side burns with long hair. My first mighty shot got him on his lower rub cage, he went staggering back surprised. With a yell he charged. Having a very long reach he caught me with a combination of punches to the head. It was my turn to stagger back; dizzy I went onto one knee. With savage glee, it was obvious he had great experience, at the intervention of the ref, he stepped back, grinning. It was the end of the boxing lesson and fighting and the last bout of the day. We all went off with our wounds to wash up for supper.

The Head Priest being as some said effeminate and avid piano player looked on in horror at our swelling condition. On enquiring to the cause of our "swellings", and on finding out, stopped the boxing "therapy" immediately. The discussions went on for a rematch in the future. Unfortunately the gloves had to be given back. Thus came to an end a seminary boxing era. As candidates for future priests, we had important decisions to make, there were pros and cons for celibacy, the church, looking after you world wide, or go out into the world and fend for yourself. Biblical arguments such as: it is not good for man to be alone, or a bird sings better with a mate, many are called, but a few are chosen. We all agreed it was a calling. Many of the boys had well to do families; they would not go on but join the family business. One went further by leaving to monastery in East Africa where one was allowed not to speak; meditation was the order of the day.

For me the writing was on the wall. I did not "fit in" I was not good at music, public speaking, acting, singing, unable to differentiate between the high notes and low notes on the priests piano, a false voice, learning the churches language Latin was beyond me. Being in self exile was not for me. I was not "called", but Providence stepped in. I failed grade 12 left. There were those who had the calling and became good and dedicated men of God, servants of the church. Some names I do remember such as: Sean Mulligan from Ireland, locals; Desmond Manheim, Richard, David, Sean an outstanding singer, Dave a portrait painter. The seminary was closed down, and converted onto an old age home, the end of another era. On a rewind or retrospect I always would wonder what type of priest I would have made out to be. Not the conventional type anyway.

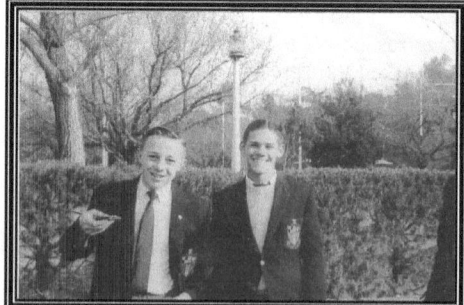

Sean Mulligan and Wally

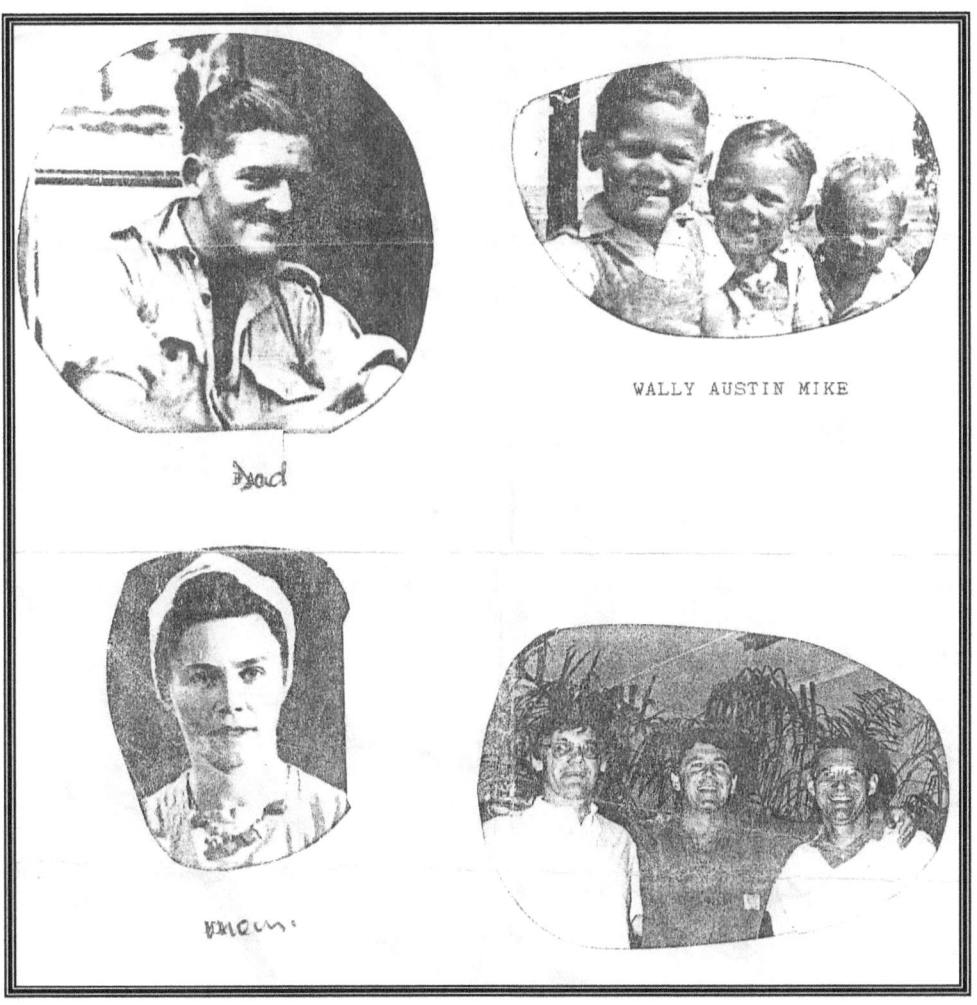

Dad

WALLY AUSTIN MIKE

Mom.

Chapter 3

Filling the gaps of time

Chapter 3   Filling the caps in time

The power of a rubber stamp

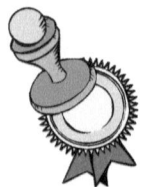

During the day while I was growing up all black people in SA had to carry Pass books, not having one on your possession meant a jail term.

From my point of view the law had to be upheld, I could see nothing wrong with caring a mere book around. Of course that was seeing from the eyes of a boy. I did hear my parents on many occasions complain about the implementation there of. The loading up suddenly any where and at any time those not having their books ready, the abuse of human rights, the abuse of power, by those wheelding it. From an early age it was drummed into me that they were inferior, a black menace, "Die Swart Gevaar", whites were in charge. The locations were situated far from the towns and at 10 o'clock a curfew would go off. It whaling in the distance would bring those not white, into action. All had to run, scamper, jog to their homes in the distant smoke and smog filled township, a place not to go to even up to today. By "Whites, bagoa" it meant literally the whites on the tops of waves as it went out to sea, obviously that name meant we had to go the same way, away from them. Their hatred was present and could be smelled. We had taken over their land and one day they would take it back, our women taken first!

In my biography I mentioned that after the seminary fiasco failing matric, and passing it at a day school in down town Johannesburg, I followed the rout of first compound work on the coal mines, a short unsuccessful attempt to get on the sea going vessels that roamed the oceans from Durban. The hard railway work there did not suit me either. From there I went to look from work in Johannesburg, Transvaal. I applied for work at the Municipality and found work as a pass control office. In my favour was knowledge of Southern Sotho, having grown up in the Eastern Free State rural area. I was quick shown the ropes of how to use the rubber stamp on pass books to control those unwanted, the raff from the homelands. Excelling at my work the bosses sent me to the troubled Soweto town ship to control the unwanted there. I did not know what was waiting for me. Having brought a JAVA 190 cc motorbike I could race to and from my home in Yeoville to work and back not depending on a poor bus service to the town ships then. I was given a small office; there the hoards came to have the right to a domicile in Johannesburg, Soweto. There long queues stretched from the said office to the pavements, a depressing sight. I had an assistant to help me; he was just as depressed as his fellows, his faith in me a round null. At head office where I had been wheelding the rubber stamp, it had been easy, cut and dried, here it was not so. The issue here was not just work related but family related. Who could live here, as decreed by law? Those born here and had documented proof had no problem, those with divided families, born in the homelands did. The forlorn faces, the hearts wrenching cries for help fell in deaf ears of the law. How could I help, I had to uphold it, not break it down.

Could I find a loop-hole to assist those in need? I did find a "gray area" to explore. There were three categories of granting permission to stay. These were namely the A, B and C permission of domicile. These were clearly marked by the by the three rubber stamps in their pass books. A was the easy decision as a birth certificate was accepted, B showing proof of 10 years of working in the area usually the pass was stamped and only required a renewal, C was the tricky one. Here the law was not very clear to any one. So I devised a plan, an opportunity did present itself quicker that I thought, to help those in need and to test the law.

A tear blackened faced hospital sister came one day after waiting in the queue for three days. She had a convincing life story. She was born and bread in Soweto, her two small children were also born there but according to tradition went to live the parents in law, a husband in Zululand. There was no documentation of their births, so they were not qualified to stay, nor was the husband a mine worker at ERPM mine. She was the only one allowed to stay, but grieving for them to stay as a family and being housed and accommodated by her work Baragwanath hospital the biggest in Africa, specializing in TB. She desperately wanted them together. With no documentation what could I do? I took a chance and asked what church she attends to and was the two children baptized there. Her answer was yes, so I told her to get the baptismal certificates as quick as possible. Plan two was that she must get her your husband to bring a letter from the mine to say he has worked there for more that 10 years. My assistant was surprised at my willingness to help; smilingly he translated my English into flawless Zulu. Happily off she went at high speed, her and her families future was in the balance. She was back that same week with all I asked her to bring. Using the powerful C rubber stamp I gave them all permission to be fully and legally domiciled in the greater Soweto. They offered me many presents of sheep and cows in thanks giving but I declined. After helping many in this way, the top management took wind of the situation and ordered me not to take such chances. A neibouring high school principal was so moved by my efforts invited me to lunch there. Eating lunch at the school and sitting under the aggressive stares of the teachers in their mass hall. When they heard the principals' story and me talking to them in there own language, they were exited to hear more of my efforts to help. Unfortunately it did not last for long, because I accepted a job on the mines for double my salary. The day I left my assistant cried like a baby. Handing in the powerful rubber stamp at head office reminded me of the rubber stamp, power over other lives, I once had, at one time in the past.

Riding Johannesburg style

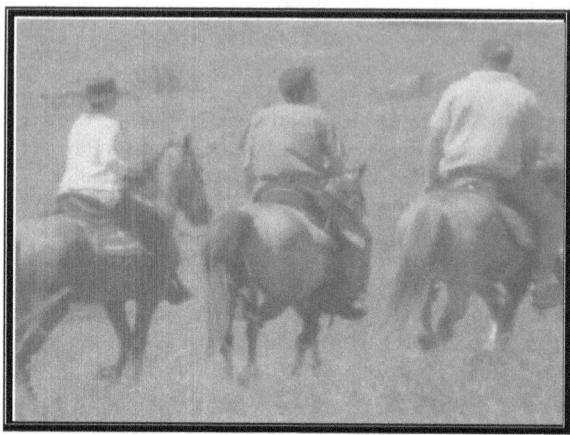

My friend, David and I were invited to spend the day at a posh riding school. The two girls who invited us were quick to tell us of all the rules and regulations governing the proper method of saddling and riding the specially fed and trained animals. No galloping or whipping the horses. All had to be ride one behind the other in single file. The club member had to ride on a go-slow walk, or go slow strike because a horse requires physical exertion by means of a strong hard gallop, to my way of thinking. Being used to fast and quick Basotho pony I was extremely frustrated and anxious to let my horse go on a gallop. I let the reins lie loose to no avail, with a light knee in the ribs, he did not want to run, was extremely fat and unfit. That was his and my undoing. Ambling under low branches, I saw my opportunity quickly I broke off a thick branch, removing the side branches and leaves. I struck my lazy Joburg horse on the rump, with a mighty crack and whip lash. More from fright than the sudden pain he broke the sound barrier galloping at a speed of an adrenalin rush, the wind in my face if felt like heaven. Three kilometers later my horse, out of breath and foaming mouth, came to a dead stop. The sweat pouring from his body, he was close to exhaustion. An hour later my girl friend came, scolding and very angry. I had violated the clubs strict code of conduct by galloping, beating a horse unnecessary which made me guilty of cruelty to animals. My excuse, I was doing the horse a favor by giving him much needed exercise was to no avail. I was mot welcome there any more and had to leave immediately. In one day I lost membership to a posh club and girl friend.

Burning floor boards

After leaving the seminary, I worked for a year at springbok colliery. It wasn't pleasant working in the black hostels. Compared to today's high standard of living and management of hostels, the living conditions were very poor. 40 workers in a room were very over crowded, strife and tension was running riot between the different black tribes.

Discipline by management was harsh, with zero tolerance. I witnessed a whipping and on completion course salt was poured on the bright red stripes across the buttocks, running with blood as they lay on the bed of punishment.

The salt in living blood, and serrated glistening buttocks coursed great pain and uncontrolled screaming, the Xhosas were voted the bravest, showing no emotion under duress. The areas around the hostels were usually covered with a thick blanket of smog from the nearby coal dumps, igniting when it rain, the stink pervaded your very being, body and clothing.

I lived in a room with a coal or wood fire place and that sparked me to leave. While out one night I came back at 2am and on opening the room door, it was engulfed by thick pungent smelling smoke, a live coal had jumped the fire and landed on the floor boards, it was now ablaze, the floor gone, now a black hole where the floor had one been, it was time for me to say goodbye to the coal mines.

A warning from above!

After burning out the floor boards of my small ex room, at Springbok Colliery it was time to move to interesting new places. Most young men would like to travel around the world. I was no exception, the Merchant navy? Where to start? Durban? A miner friend of mine had trouble with a jealous husband, so we decided after too much brandy mixed with Lion lager to leave as soon as possible, his life at stake. The village rumor had it that the husband had a double barreled shot gun; ready to shoot him where it hurt.

"Kom engelsman, kom ons maak gat skoon, ek wil nie kennis maak met hael patrone nie. Ek is te jonk om nou dood te gaan vir 'n skelm knippie."

Before the sun came up the next morning we were both halfway to the sea. His faded green Beatle Volkswagen slowly groaned and roared over the winding Drakensberg pass, where the British red coats were cut down by the more accurate firepower of the Boers. Obviously the English had to change from bright red, not an un-missable target to khaki, hence the name khaki boer.

Durban: A flying hot rod

We both got work at Durban Railways, me as a carriage demolisher. The professional who knew his job took two days to cut up the iron carriage into pieces until the 4 wheels were left. It took me one day to remove one very rusty bolt, and that same bolt fell into my glasses. When asking the foreman for the day off to get new spectacles he was very unhappy. I was transferred the next day to the workshops, where they made railway carriage springs or shock absorbers.

I landed at the blacksmith shop. Here 2m flat bars red hot after coming out of the furnace were bent by being struck in the center with a heavy 14lb hammer. It looked easy enough to do. "Take a shot" said the foreman. Hefting the hammer above my head, aiming, with all my strength I let fly. The hammer head, flowing in arc, struck the side of the bar with a mighty twang. The rod spun away towards a bunch of fellow workers nearby, looking like a bright red rocket in its flight to its landing place. The hot rod landed between the legs of the foreman, from behind. There ensured a deathly silence. The burning of human flesh could be smelled; the overall flames could be seen. A loud painful scream was heard, "Wally I am going to kill you" is all I heard. I dropped the hammer and fled.

Another foreman gave me an easier safer job cutting 12 inch rods with a angle grinder. His instructions were "work safer, keep away from the other workers, and wear your safety goggles and near safety leather gloves. You are an accident about to happen. "

Weekends I went swimming on Durban's beaches and relaxed. My aim to go around the world had not diminished. At every opportunity I was at her harbor to chat to the sea going ships captains. At that time it was most difficult to obtain a SA passport, those belonging to the US or Britain was acceptable only.

Durban's plans did not materialize. All fell to nothing, a waste of time.

My friend I never saw, he drinking and womanizing his life away. I decided being extremely lonely, to go home to my family in Johannesburg. I booked a flight from Durban homeward bound.

Durban was a mistake, it was only a place to relax and have a holiday, not work!

I was very excited to go on my first flight on a Boeing 707!

My first flight

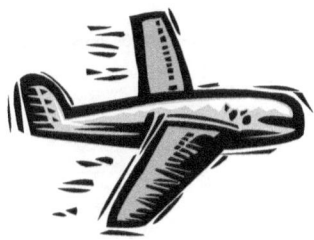

When my great expectations as young man to get a passport, travel the wide oceans by ship came to nothing, I felt dejected and hopeless, life without a purpose. I resigned from the Durban railways and looked worth, to family in Johannesburg may be other work? Transport was the problem. It was 600 miles away one the Drankensberg Range of high mountains. Too get there, by bus, too boring, by air, yes, exiting, a new experience awaited.

I booked a fight to Jan Smuts, Johannesburg at the travel agency in Durban. A bus took me to the air terminal, I was very excited! My first flight! At the long queue we boarded the great plane. Soon we were strapped down. The Air Hostess gave us a long lecture on what to do in a case of emergency. Soon the planes engines ignited with a deafening roar! The plane was moving! With a slight jerk we had a lift off! As we emerged away from Durban I could see to the east the sea stretching, a long expanse of deep blue, it was disappeared as we turned away and rose higher and higher into the air. We swept above the clouds at high speeds. Far below the great Darkensberg was only seen by a smudge of green lines. No towns could be seen. "Please, fasten your seat belts" the Air hostess said. It felt like moments before when we left Durban! We were now over Johannesburg. From the air it looked awesome! A giant web of roads and buildings, stretching in all directions!

We landed with a thump. The wheels striking the air strips fast, the breaks giving a screeching sound. We were safely landed! It felt like a dream, one moment in Durban in its sweltering heat, the next in Gauteng in less that an hour. They call it "jet lag" Taking a bus I was met with open arms at my parent's home, at that time Mike was at Universality and Aussie at Standard Bank. I quickly found work at Johannesburg municipality as a Pass control Officer.

My first Car

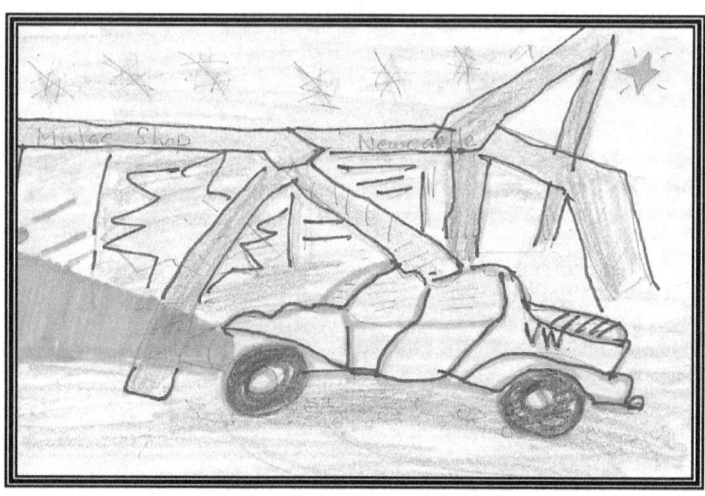

Being a learner miner and earning R90.00 per month was difficult, but to try and save for a car was asking too much. First off all my friends were all heavy drinkers and spent their free time at the mine club where the alcohol was cheaper. Being a loner by nature I did not join in their merriment, especially at month end to celebrate pay day. After three months of saving I had the necessary R300.00 deposit. While my fellow learners were playing ball on the rugby field I arrived with my shiny white Volkswagen Sedan not the beatle shape. They could not believe I now owned a car. "Where did I get the money from?" They asked. The car and I were the center of attraction. I really loved to drive and listen to the roar and beat of the engine. I used to drive to a friend from school days, his name also Walter, to a town called Newcastle in Natal. We were altar boys years back. Unfortunately on that weekend we drank too much cane and sprite a favorite to Natalian's then. Being a top rally driver he took over the wheel that was a mistake I would later regret. The timing was bad it was just passed midnight the town streets quiet. With a Volkswagens roar we took short cuts through prominent citizens rose gardens. Their house lights went on, they called the police but we were long gone, our drunken laughter echoing over the hill where we sat on the rocks finishing off the bottle. We would race through town with its one main street and tell the cops to go to hell. Our descent from the hill to town was fast, very fast. The adrenalin was pumping at full blast and so was the cane, the speedometer showed 140 km/ph. Recklessly we roared into the town. Going into a broadside, slipping on loose gravel and oil we rocketed straight into an Indian general store. The front of the car cut off the three poles keeping up the front roof. We careened into the shop and came to a dead and sudden stop. The car now a mangled wreck and the shop roofless with groceries all over we sat there mesmerized. Stunned, my head was bleeding, but Walter was unscathed laying on the pavement in a daze. Much trouble awaited us the police who were looking for us, the Indian shopkeeper was in a rage, he was taking us to court. That was the sorry end of my first and most lovely car. My girlfriend Martie, now my wife, was not amused at all.

Hillbrow: The accident 1965

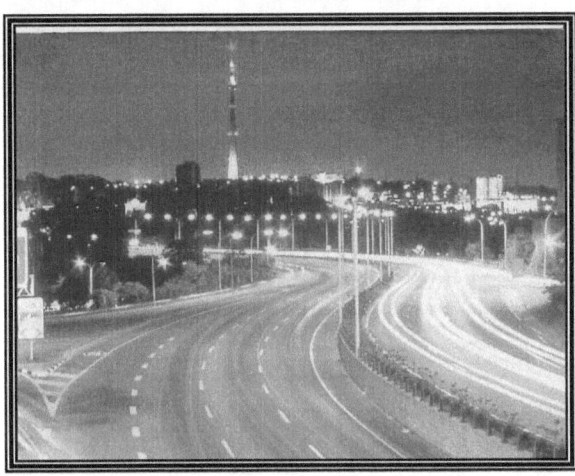

It was Hillbrow at its worst, peak hour traffic at six. The Joberg workers were on their way home. All traffic was popping out of high flying garages, car ports and streets where they had stood for the day. All traffic lights, controlling this bed-lam of thousands of vehicles con verging on them, Hillbrow the main exit and bottle neck.

Standing on the side street you could smell the exhaust smoke with its chocking gasses, the Soweto smog was also creeping up, a pungent odour of its own, a result of a thousand fires stocking up for supper, their black owners in jam packed busses heading there anticipation, salivers dripping.

After work, computers were tired, small incidents of traffic hogging like cutting you off or hooting from behind would bring on a rage, at the present time called "road rage". The city lights had just come on, a disgruntled black uniformed cop was directing traffic at a broken down robot intersection, his white gloved hands gesticulating, controlling the traffic flow, he had the power to stop any vehicle, no matter how big or small with a lift of one white gloved hand!

Those were the 1960's, a far cry when it came to safety at night in the city. I could walk with out any fear from the city center to the notorious Hillbrow, at that time, a white residential area. Only on one day of the year no one would venture there was on New Years night, your car would be scrapped by hooligans, with new years fever out of control, a chaos of curses and yells.

Back at the "ranch" 82 Georges street, I had just got on to my Java 190, and with spinning back wheels and grinding gears I was on the way to the city center, my destination the Johannesburg Municipal Gym. I was late my big weight training partner would be waiting impatiently for me.

I had a very bad habit of timing the speedy jaw so as to pass the robots when they turned green, in the distance they would be red, with out gearing down or losing speed. It was a game of adrenalin pump, a surging excitement; one mistake would mean a crash, hospital admittance. After turning off from Jan Smuts avenue, it would mean cutting through Hillbrow. In the distance the robots colour was a deep red, to the left of me was the SAP Police Station, ahead the said robot beaconing me to come faster. It was on a hill and I past through the intersection at speed, the light had turned a dark green, the rider and bike had made it with milliseconds to spare, or so I thought. Below the grade line of the said robot was a stop street; here an impatient driver of a Ford also took his chance to get to his destination quicker. He was a doctor at the Provincial hospital in his way to attend to patients, he would also become one. In front of me loomed his white car, suddenly in my path. There was no time to brake; I connected him "broadside". By a miracle, I on impact flew over the white bonnet, upside down, as if time stood still, I remember up to this day those bright stars blinking high in the heavens, blackness above.

By another miracle I landed uninjured on the palm of my left hand, a slight swelling resulted. Not so with my doctor friend, he had banged his forehead badly against the windscreen in a shatter. Jumping up I ran to his aid. Being a medical man he had in his cubby hole a first aid kit with bandages, this I quickly used to wrapped his bleeding head, when the bleeding had stopped and he feeling better he rounded on me calling me names and that he would see me in court for negligent driving.

Luckily for him he could start his Ford and go to work. My transport on the other hand had a flattened front wheel, its body now in the shape of a bent branch, never to recover its former self. I had to drag it with pouring oil and running petrol over the tar road, out of the way of the now traffic jam. As mentioned the SAP wasn't far from the robot. Here I gave my account of the accident. "The Ford's driver had jumped the stop sign, I was not the guilty one." The sergeant only gave me a knowing smile. I hopped on a bus, my gym and training out of my mind naturally after the shock. A friend of mine from England sold me his Zuzuki 500cc, a faster and bigger bike. I was told by mail that I, was not needed at the enquiry as the good doctor, being on a 24 hour day had no time to report the incident, he was founded guilty in abstentia of not stopping at that stop sign, I was Scott free.

It is needless to say that I did become more careful, avoiding that "roll in the air" during peak time traffic and slowing down at or near robots. Today Hillbrow is no different; peak period is a time slot, and place to be avoided at all costs like a dreaded disease.

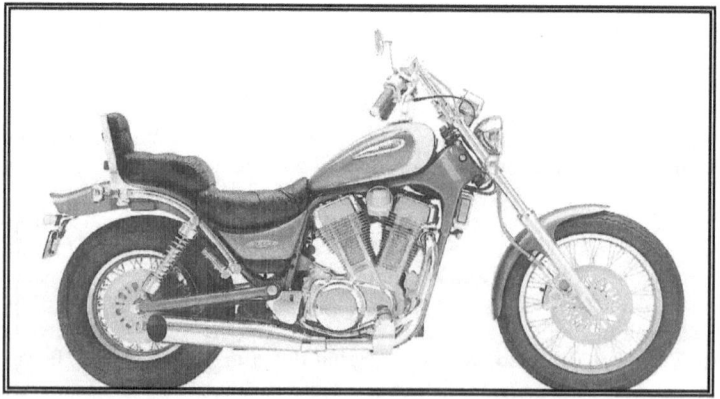

When fishing is not fishing – 1970

As a pass- control officer in Soweto, Johannesburg, I left behind an atmosphere of conflict. This came about because of the conflict of interests, resulting from the strict enforcement of the act that said where black people should live. The "power that were" reasoned that if they did not qualify for residence then they should go back to their ancestral home, "in the mountains" as it were. These homes were far from the Metropolis of now, Gauteng. The unwanted came illegally from the Basotho highlands, the coastlands of the Transkei and Zululand valley of a thousand hills. Especially these chiefs and head men did not like their young men and women leaving, as their life style of tribalism and tradition would be destroyed.

The godless way of the while mans money, alcoholism, prostitutes, anti tribalism, anti chief, and anti authorities there for their own eventual demise would result. The world acclaimed book, "Cry the beloved country" a good example of that break-down, as early as 1946. What both sides forgot was the food and hunger situation of their people, no certain traditions or rules to sustain them. Mitigating factors were poor methods of black farming such as, overgrazing, no land rotation of crops, left a rid desert behind. Another example was the indiscriminate use of trees for winter fires, the nightly pungent odour of the listlessly hanging smoke as a foggy blanket as it were, over the locations, were a reflection of where the trees went.

So in this unhappy and unhealthy atmosphere, the mighty flow of migrant labour started, Gauteng, "the place of gold" the main attraction. The sprawling shanty towns of Soweto started. Today the situation is worsened by loss and lack of work. These "plakker" have spread like a diseased cancerous virus over the whole of South Africa. Even a peaceful holiday town like Jefferysbay has had to build kilometers of high walls around properties for protection. As mentioned I left the Witwatersrand and home to start a new career as a miner in the now Mpumulanga, the Evander gold fields. At that time there were just open velds where the mighty Sasol now stands.

O arrived at the Government Miners training college to be signed on a learner miner, the work seekers started at my mode of transport, a bent back(after the accident in Hillbrow) Java 190cc. In our class were five-teen learners, mostly from stock, ready to make money. We were issued with a round silver railway watch to be kept in a leather belt pouch, the other clothes were mine boots, gloves, overalls and a safety mine helmet.

We became super fit doing all the manual work, and preparing for the qualification of mine blasting ticket and then becoming miners where the big money was. The routine was basically to work like a dog, eat like a pig, muscle for power, drink like a fish and sleep like tired lambs. For recreation we either played the popular sport of rugby or enjoyed the quiet waters of the dam fishing.

This is where my story comes in.

That weekend when the boys ere talking excitedly about the many fishing spots around the area of Kinross, nearby. I was amazed at the tonnage of fish brought back, either eaten over the coals or sold at the locations, the hungry glad to have high protein food to replace the day to day "pap".

I did not have my own transport, so I had to go along with a boisterous group in a beat up Toyota bakkie1600. We packed the car with plenty of Klifdrift and coke. In a corner was a hold on satchel with "bread" in it for the fishing hooks, which I did not see, or rods fro that matter. That was strange. I was soon to find out what the "bread" was, DYNAMITE. Once the company of revelers had settled down to some serious drinking the fun started. "Pass op boys" the shout went up. High in the sky with a great loop, thrown by hand, went the short fused "bomb" when off, a meter below the wavy surface of the once tranquil dam. After the concussion had done its job thirty big fish came suddenly to the surface, dead and floating. With cries of the hunter the fishermen collected the "booty" by netting them out. The fire had been going strongly, the savoury dishes put carefully into foil paper, and the boys were past masters.

In our excitement we did not notice or see the owner of the dam arriving at high speed, he had heard the boom of the illegal fishing methods and was going to put a stop to it immediately. He was driving a well worn Beatle, Volkswagen car, the leader of our group having experience of such "tight" situations, let out a yell to warn everyone, "los alles en spring in die bakkie, vinnig!" (Leave everything and jump into the car, now!)

With a sudden twist of the wrist, and turning around at speed just like a Springbok cricket bowler, they threw the weapon at the on coming farmers as if at war. With a fast sprint for his life our leader dived into the roaring waiting "bakkie" at high speed and urgency its back wheels spinning, clumps of grass churned up, the bakkie was enrooted for the getaway. A muffled roar erupted under the chasing Beatle. The power of the blast lifted it meters high off the ground. It somersaulted twice in the air and remarkably landed like a circus act on its now flat and burst tyres. We were at that stage only worried about our getting away safely and not so much concerned about the big angry farmers' health.

The evidence of fish was thrown out along the way. The black people along the gravel roads were too happy to find fish hurled at them, it was their supper! Arriving at the college we quickly cleaned the bakkie, put our mine clothing on and headed for the nearby shaft to do some unexpected overtime. A turbaned farmer did come the next day only to find on one to answer his angry questions. In black mood he went back to his farm to await our return, a long three meter shambuk in hand, we never went back.

Bad Breath

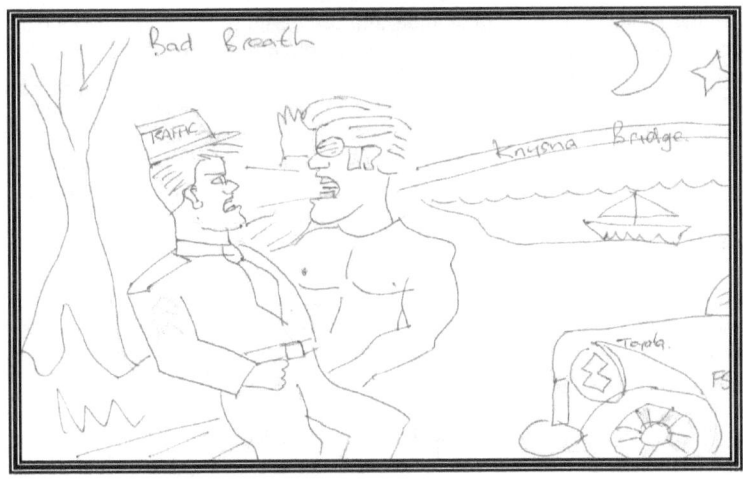

My wife, Martie complained day and night about my bad breath. She could not live with it or me anywhere near her. It stank of rotten carrion. Using all types of mouth washes, toothpastes and brushes to try to clear the smell, it did not help and was to no avail.

Eventually on this crises situation I went to the dentist and his prognosis was: back drip of the throat. He gave me a course of antibiotics to follow. He also installed a set of false teeth similar to braces for the lower set. To not have examined them, and telling me they were in a good condition and not to remove them unless necessary would be proved later to be his undoing. Being short of money at that time, and being behind with the house bond payment, I received an offer of employment. My son in law, Safry had a recycling bottle business in Knysna 1000 km away from Welkom, and I accepted.

The job entailed going into the black and brown townships, to collect old cold drink, brandy, gin and cane bottles to be resold for a profit. On Mondays after the weekends was when the bakkie became overloaded. We were making a living out of other peoples bad and thirsty alcoholic drinking habits.

On certain Saturday night at about midnight Safry called me by phone, saying in a incoherent manner that he had drunk too much and that I should come and fetch him. To make matters worse he warned me that on the way to the club on the exit bridge of Knysna were traffic officers doing a road block. Chancing that, he would spend the week end in the "slammer", he was therefore unfit to drive home.

My 'beat up' Corolla was also unfit for the road. It had no brakes, had only one headlight working and so to fetch him would be suicide, but I was prepared to go to the rescue. My plan was to drive, but to stick as closely as possible to the car in front of me, so as to avoid detection by the waiting speed cops on the bridge. Luckily I attached myself to a new "Merc", on crossing the bridge the traffic officials knowing him let him through with a friendly wave of the hand. Seeing me, a junk car behind the new one, they waved me down to stop. I did not. Their shouts and curses could be heard behind as I accelerate away. At the end of the bridge I swerved to right and shot under the bridge. There I found an unsteady Safry, he had also heard the commotion as the speed cops with their blue and red flashing lights, hot in pursuit and were getting closer fast. I spun the Toyota to the nearest clump of trees out of reach and Saf followed. The two traffic officials came, their cars roaring, brakes skidding, headlights pointing at us and then came to a sudden stop in front of us. Getting out at speed the men in uniform approached us, me standing at Saf's bakkie. "Who is the driver of that fucked up Toyota?" the first official asked in a shout. They were like two bullterriers! I am I answered as if nothing was wrong. "You nearly ran me over!" he screamed in a babble of anger. "Why didn't you stop?" his voice now a horse whisper. "You are drunk and I want to check the alcohol content of your breath!" breathing in my face now.

Obligingly and obediently I let him have a lung full of my best non-alcoholic breath, the same breath my wife was complaining about for so long. Taking in the breath he breathed in the foul air, he staggered back. "I smell no liquor on you," he muttered incoherently, gasping for fresh air in the night wind, coming off the Knysna Lake.

Perplexed at the unexpected bad smell never before smelled from a live person he was non-pulsed on what to do next. Safry came to the rescue, explaining why I was there in the firs place. Admitting to having too much drinks to himself fed by his many admiring tipsy listeners enhanced also by his tear jerking love songs.

Knowing him as the local celebrity they relaxed and accepted his explanation of his father in law coming to fetch him in his hour of need. With many warnings and admonishing they left disgustedly. Later at home with Angie, my daughter heavily pregnant with their first child, we celebrated with a good laugh.

Back in Welkom, my mouth now in intolerable pain, I went to another dentist. He looked on in horror at my now nearly putrefied mouth condition. Donning his face mask he took out the stinking false teeth. I explained that the former dentist did not allow me to remove them; he was not amused at all at this information. His instructions were to wash them daily and before coming back, to go on to antibiotics.

The source of the terrible hyena breath was now solved. My mouth was now back to normal, and so was my love life. The bad breath saga was now as said, solved for good.

Kentucky Fried Chicken 2000

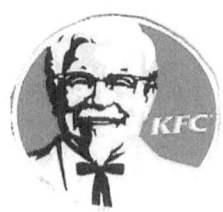

After the mine accident and recuperating fast, I felt I had to go to work; sitting at home vegetating wasn't for me. Some incidents I do remember of how I felt, being at home thankfully; out of hospital, but trying to get to grips with my broken body. Before the accident I was a regular gym guy, going to a well equipped gym, called Kiewiet's Gym. Here Quintin, my son and I spent hours pumping iron. I weighed in at a healthy and strong weight of 90 kg. According to the Doctors I would not have seen the light of day if my body was in a poor and untrained shape.

I will always remember with fondness and appreciation those who took time off to visit me. The light at ICU was always in dim so I could not know the time of day. Martie was a regular visitor, exerting me to get up and go. She even organized the staff to sing. They gathered around my bed and sang the most melodious songs, to me sounding rapture from heaven. No better therapy for the spirit. Lillian my eldest daughter always made time to see me during her lunch break from the town library, bringing sweets and cold drink. I also thank the rest of the family for their undying support. On discharge the relief of coming out was too much, seeing the sun, hearing the birds chirping. I cried like a new born, sobbing with relief.

At home I was trying to get used to the hated wheel-chair, my legs being inactive for three months, they were too weak for normal walking. A month later I was walking with a walker, a month later with two crutches, a month later one crutch, then very wobbly, weakly and slowly then faster too both feet and legs. It took me a full year to recuperate. Those days of training with small weights and the whole body shacking like a drunken were over, I felt better. On one of my visits to the specialist, he examined me for workman's compensation; he suggested I go to the psychiatrist so as to work through the past traumatic experience of the mine accident. He said that my bones would mend but more importantly were the scares, unseen, left behind on the spirit, mind and soul. Talking to the psychiatrist would benefit me tremendously. I went the "visit". To my surprise she was not only a beautiful and charming Doctor but a woman who knows her job. We had met before, she coming to me at my lowest, at ICU.

She explained that after being through a traumatic experience, it was advisable to go back to the scene and as it were to relive it, and conquer those demands nagging at your subconscious. His job was to reveal to me as a therapy, through a process of revealing the subconscious, inducing me to relate with out rest details of the accident and to go beyond that to earlier life's experiences. She was an expert, talking softly in a bed side manner, coxing me to talk. Her objective was to detect hidden mental conflicts which if not detected would produce disorders in my mind. Knowing them, she would be able to treat them by telling them to me, and so in my turn be treated mentally. My wife, Martie was already complaining that I was a different man to the one who had gone into the hospital. We joked about it saying I had received so many blood transfusions, that I had the blood and personalities of many, not my own. I spoke with out restraint, her interest in my past growing. I had been in a Roman Catholic seminary. There were many devils I had to fight. At one stage I was fasting and doing penance, part of the penance was to walk with small stones in my shoes; this would drive away bad thoughts, and bring punishment to myself, self inflicted. Another method was to wrap around my tummy a, what we call "blou-draad" or wire. The excruciating pain around the midriff would make me pure so that I could be worthy of a dedicated priest. Going back even further into my past, she heard that I was molested at an early age by our black maid. I was walking around with this guilt to long, it was not my fault!

The hypnotic therapy, as it were, changed my perspective of looking at my self, I had to accept, looking ahead and get on with my life, self recrimination was the worst thing to have nagging all the time. She explained that not controlled would lead to break down and so mending of the spirit, in extreme cases self torment could lead to suicide. I was a man getting better. The nightmare was over, the mind and body had to get back to a higher level of healthiness.

We knew very good friends the Van Der Walts who offered me work as a 5 ton lorry driver. I went to work for them. The work entailed transporting acetylene and oxygen bottles to clients all over the Welkom area. I enjoyed the driving, but the lifting of the heavy iron cylinders was back breaking. At times I also assisted as a store man, some times filling up gas bottles and helping with the office and computer entries. Answering the phone and being a general help.

Driving the lorry, loading and off loading brought me to some time in Johannesburg. After a hard days work my assistant and I turned off to have a tasty meal as we were hungry. We found a suitable place Kentucky Fried Chicken, the whole area was filled with hordes of people coming and going. There were so many people pushing and shoving. I left my assistant in the lorry, locked up so that he would not be hijacked. Having brought watering tasty and succulent chicken, I strolled out of the shop. With one hand holding the packet of chicken pieces for the assistant, the other in my mouth, there is no other chicken that draws the tongue and chewing motion into that tasty chicken. Deep in thought I limped slowly, still not fully recovered, intent on getting back, I did not notice three hoodlums stealthily approaching me, me being a "soft target". With lightning speed they attacked. One had a sharp knife to my throat; I still remember vividly how I was going to land up in hospital, blood pouring from that knife wound.

Now fully paralyzed from shock, standing like a cement statue, the other hoodlum cut, expertly the bean bag off my waist. The third crook held me fastened, his sweaty arms around my waist, his breath stinking of stale cigarettes and" kaffir" beer. This all took place in a matter of seconds. Suddenly letting go they ran like hounds, in thee different directions. I could not even yell or shout, but the tasty morsel was still in my mouth blocking any attempted sound or utterance. Dejected I could only walk back to the assistant and relate the harrowing tale to him. Having been brought up in the township this wasn't a surprise for him.

On reporting the incident to the SAP, it was such a common occurrence to them that nothing could be done. At least I had done my duty. There are two things I am wary of, first wearing bean bags, a potential soft target for a thief, and secondly the day when Kentucky Fried Chicken was so delicious I lost track of my surroundings for a moment.

Chapter 4
Married life

Chapter 4   Married life

Martie and Wally

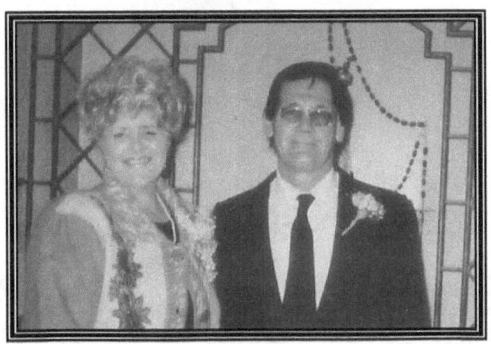

To get married may not seem difficult, but in my case it was. The first problem was that when the Nederlands Gerformeerde Kerk heard that Martie Coetzee a member of their church was getting married to a Roman Catholic, she was expelled immediately, with out a hearing. My family was opposed to my marriage to an Afrikaner. They in turn opposed a marriage to an Englishman. For three years Martie and I fought for our rights. We won the battle and got married with every ones blessings. We got married in Evander where she and her family lived. The candle lit ceremony impressed my Father in law. After the wedding vows and get together, we left for Durban. Our honeymoon was fantastic and unforgettable. I was in love!

Martie would become a catholic later; I worked in Bloemfontein as a branch manager for a shoe company, but would go back to the mines as they had maternity benefits and cheaper housing. We moved to Welkom there I started to work on the gold mines. We stayed in a flat, and there our first born Lillian was born, followed by Charlotte, Quintin our first son, then Angelique came lastly Patrick was born. Our union brought five blessed and healthy children. The many medal and trophies adorning show case bear witness to the fact. Lillian and Charlotte broke records at school with athletics, year after year. Quintin achieved Springbok Colours for chess in the junior school. Quintin and Patrick, the age of five, were competing nation wide in BMX racing. Later Lillian took part in Modeling and Angelique excelled at ballet. The rest of us did Karate together. Patrick the youngest won his Springbok with Tae Kwondo. He represented South Africa in London. He excelled himself further by winning the cover title of Mr. Junior South Africa in a nation wide modeling competition, his site on a modeling contract overseas. My beautiful wife was a champion pistol shot, beating many men at their own game, including myself. They all went to school in Welkom, blessed with good health, passed Grade 12, and went out to work. The fruit of our marriage we were happy blessing. Of course many grand children followed, the happiness and blessing have not stopped.

Charlotte's two children are too adorable, they are Tistan and Tyran. There Grandmother loves to spoil them when ever we get a change to visit them. The entire family is exceeding exceptionally well with Karate. Both Charlotte and Nico her husband have got black belt in Karate. Their two precious children will definitely follow, when you see them copying their parents Karate moves.

When the Welkom Girds go on a picnic

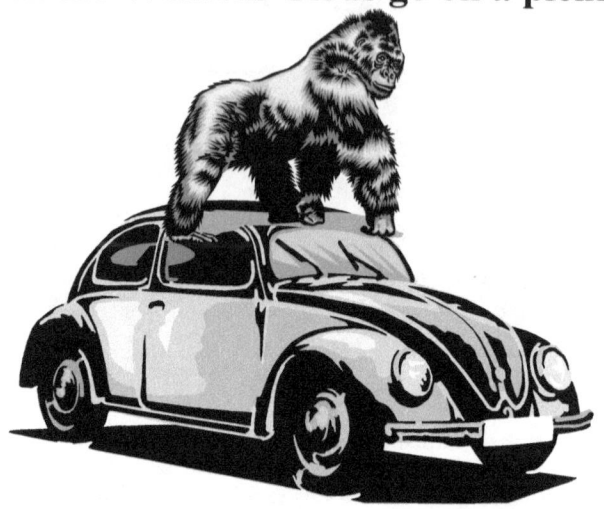

Where we went for a outing was a place called then, Willem Pretorius Nature Reserve. It is situated between a town called Ventersburg and Windburg. At that time there were no tarred roads on the reserve itself. From the main highway it twisted and turned, angling between and directly past the great Allemanskraal high dam wall shimmering under the direct sun light when the small and tiny water droplets ran directly down its brown and yellow faded concrete, holding back that accumulated mass of dirty brown rain water, behind it. Around this dam are small elongated hills in a bow shaped to assist in the water flow from the higher level when it rained in the summer months.

As you explore this region of scenic tapesterial beauty and its soul touching stillness and tranquility its almost overwhelming in its power of natural magnetisms, a life of its own. To the east lies majestic mountains with sandstone serrated yellow perpendicular cliffs, farms not seen, only by that mighty eagle flying lazily just below the wisp of a cloud, also not seen by us were the outstretched fields of cosmos, the golden hues of sun flowers. Many small and larger dams are dotted around, increasing in number and as the Easter Free State emerges, the soil for maize, fertile.

Nearby is the much acclaimed and famous Golden Gate National Park described in another chapter. One thing we don't thing about ere the bygone wars, between black on black or white against white, their foot prints as it were left behind through their memorials, spent rifle cartridges. I found many of these on the Black Mountain, called Thaba Nchu. At this park is also the site of small rock made igloos, a past prehistoric area, fossil foot prints not seen by us laymen, are hidden. Sand stone buildings in abundance are built as a distinctive feature of each town, sand stone churches, of unequalled quality, mainly due to its mode of construction lovingly land crafted. Each stone a work of art, in honour of God? To come back to our picnic story at this reserve, its inhabitants many types of wild animals, from baboons to rhinos, birds and snakes we drove through.

Our motor car was a yellow coloured Volkswagen beatle shape, a car to rely on. In it were myself, Martie, Lillian and Charlotte, the other three children to come, not yet born.

At a top of a single fitted hill we stopped, and got out here the "padkos" was taken out of the boot of the car situated in front, the large multi-coloured Basotho blanket was spread out of the soft green grass, the feast at hand, the children expectantly hungry. We all ate the boere wors, freshly backed bread, boiled eggs and jam; we were all in a good mood enjoying the outing, the wonderful scenery. When we finished our lunch, the energy of the children took over. They explored the surroundings, minds alert to natures beauty.

Above us were a school of baboons, watching us. May be they were hungry and also wanted to join in our picnic? To describe the largest of them, the powerful leader, would be as follows: his muzzle was elongated like a dog's, strong canine teeth glinted in the sun rays. Its tail was short, nails also short, cheeks pouched, blackened, weather beaten. His eyes were small, back, sharp, cruel and deep set. The eye brows fluffy huge, his back side was reddish in colour, naked callosities in the hips, a master baboon, to be feared.

Having had our fun we were now on our way home, but would first see the wild animals, with the well known roar of the engine at the back we pulled away. A the next bend on the dirt road we came face to face with our friend just described, a mirthless smile, a smirk to welcome us! Surrounding him were others, of different sizes, females with their shrilly crying babies in their backs, many child baboons scampering around in attendance. Our large friend and family had smelled the food just eaten and were now expectant of some for themselves.

Suddenly with a mighty inhuman leap our blood shot eyed hairy friend landed on the roof of the small car with a thud. The vehicle nearly tipped over with the force of the landing. We were terrified, helpless we all screamed as in one voice. The intruder sat fixed on top, his calloused hands and dirty smelling feet gripped the side of the doors. Accelerating the car, suddenly stopping so as to topple him off, were to no avail. We were struck in a giant monster's vice. His back side red, and tail hung over the side, His one eye was watching us from above through the wind screen, he was enjoying this cat and mouse death game, and we weren't.

On an impulse, Martie took hold of a pair of sharp scissors used for dress making, she being a past master at it. Driving this weapon with a heave and mighty upward force, it entered the buttocks of our friend, the leader of the hungry pack! The sharp serrated point on entering the muscle, bone, and marrow causing a terrible reaction to erupt from the slimy red mouth.

The whole car shook, the great predator was in a fury, the pain too much. The blood and excreta flowing down along side the car, the shock of Marties attack too much. At that moment I accelerated away, now off balance he rolled away in a ball of grey fur, a bloody mess. We were free! This incident must have taken a few minutes but for us the time was slow, elongated, a painful memory, but a fortunate one, where a baboon saw his ass! Relieved we got back to our home in Welkom in one piece!

A strong person

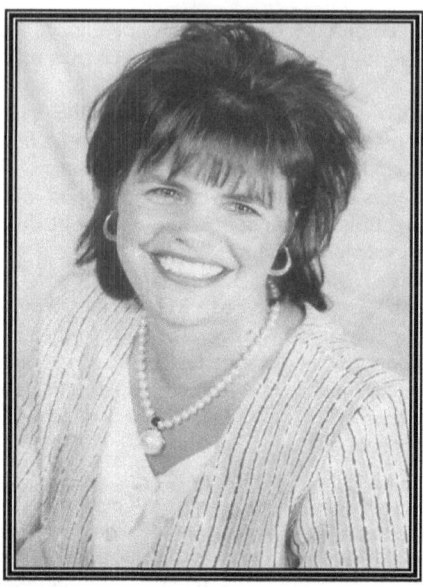

Some people are born to go though more hardships than others. Through their hardships they become stronger and more confident. That inner power takes over, that spirit is then manifest. They themselves can't see it but we on the other side can. A major problem can rear its ugly head but you will only hear of it later when it had been solved even at a price. She is that person. This person's attitude is her essence. The opposite to that of the evil one breaking down not building up, her essence is love and understanding. She went through much suffering when he second born son fell inadvertently into their shallow swimming pool. The event was fatal and tragic. Luckily and through fate she has a strong husband to rely on, a man among men, Hannes.

She is inseparable from her elder's son Walter, always a helping hand. Her name is Maureen Lillian my eldest daughter the co-editor of the narrative. Thank you. She was given a second chance. A beautiful daughter was born, her third child. His parting filled the sorrowful 'leaving' of small Tiaan. Crystal by name is just that, a jewel, a shinning example of a strong, clever and healthy girl.

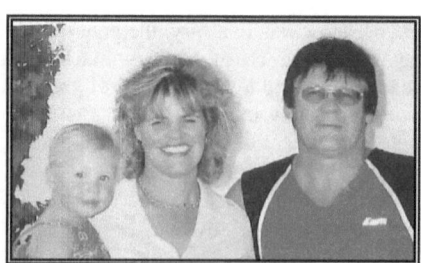

The leader of the pack

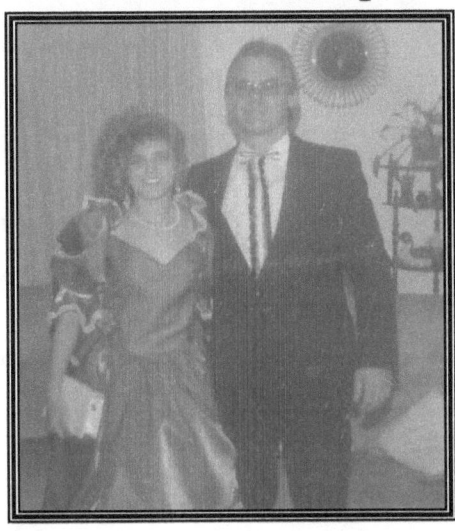

She came into the world sliding as it were on caster oil. Martie's mother gave her advice that if the period of nine months was over, then the baby must come, even with out its permission, drinking caster oil before the event, to speed its coming quicker and faster. Martie did what her mother said, and drank the oil, at seven that night, but at nine while in the hot bath those painful contractions came in a series, suddenly.

"Get the car ready, and the bag, our son is on his way" shouted Martie. At Welkom provincial hospital there was no time for the usual inspections of the mother, she was rushed at full speed, abdomen in the air, to the Maternity ward. I did the pushing of the bed trolley. On arriving at the door I was told to stand out side it would be a difficult delivery and fathers usually faint or interfered when their dear wives screamed.

I stood alone in the long hospital corridor, I didn't ask why but the passage was pitch black and dark. In that darkness and quietness a signal piecing mother scream punctured the still black night. What followed was that well known heart rending new born baby's whail. At that moment any where in the world in the same situation people's emotion runs away, the cry with joy. A new person has arrived out of the Xmas box. I was no exception, the tears flowed, and happiness paramount, my second child was born.

This occasion a reminder, of two years previously when our first born came. I was a miner busy supervising work being done; the Shift Boss arrived out of breath to tell me the good news. The cage was organized and while running to the station in the darkened tunnels, the cap lamp lighting a few meter a head, the tears flowed down my cheeks.

I WAS A FATHER, THE GREATEST GIFT IN THE WORLD" sobbing with joy I arrived at the cage, the bells were rung and away I was whisked. The gigantic pull of the cage pressure was felt, as it ascended to surface. I felt every bump and heard every rickety sound as the cage was propelled upwards. The flashing of the levels or different stations rushed past. I was the happiest day of my life, not counting my Wedding Day of course.

Now the second bundle of joy had arrived, I standing in the dark, mesmerized with emotion. A Dr Bonnett arrived at high speed, my daughter Chartlotte was faster, she had arrived before the good doctor could even lift a finger. The sister in charge was there, it was a piece of cake for her. He lifting the baby by its feet, upside down, a smart smack on the back, the bronchial tubes open, the new born would give its customary gugle sound, like the grand entrance of a queen.

Charlotte was different to her sister; she cried a lot, we finding out that she was allergic t milk, so remained stunted and small. This was not a handicap by any means. She was "supposed to be a boy", and made for that as she grew up. No boy was a match for her when it came to climbing, running and speed. At the Convent where she went to school, no record stood, when she challenged it. She was the most successful athlete produced by them. To make a point she would race against girls twice her size and win by ten meters.

At school in the class she was the leader of the pack. She had a huge following of admires, but her leadership skills would be tested, with those very admires on a mountain at the Golden Gate National Park, in the Easter Free State.

I was the driver of one of the three school buses to take them to the park. Leaving early that morning for the journey the girls were like kinder garden children on their first hike, laughing and chatting, looking foreword to the outing.

Golden Gate National Park: Easter Free State

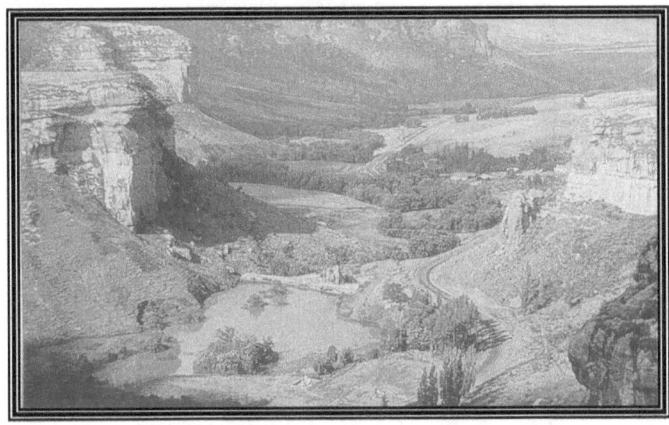

This park nestles at the foot of the great Maluties, home to many varieties of mammals, like the black wildebeest, eland, blesbok, oribi, springbok, zebras, many birds including the bearded vulture. The ibis (dassie) and the rare but bald kind bred on the ledge of the steep stand stone cliffs. They could look out to the picture of breath taking nature tapestry of different colours of hues, red, yellow, purple, green and orange all shades merging and mingling making it a picture drawn in heaven. Towards evening the sun setting is spectacular in its smoldering like colours, different hues of red and purple fading into the night, only to be repeated the following grand day. The moon would then take over as a smiling silent partner.

This park derives its name from the brilliant shades of gold cast by that sun on the sand stone cliffs, given that magnetic effect on the viewer. The largest of these is called the Brand Wag rock or sentinel, keeping watch and keeping vigil over man and beast under its rule, as it were.
On arriving at the park described the Convent girls with Charlotte at the head, were quickly organized and dressed to go steep cliff climbing. Soon you could see the mountaineers, now a thin line looking like army ants, winding there way to the top. You could hear their joys, shouting and yelling, the echoes vibrating from cliff to cliff. I, on the other had been too slow, but come from behind as a rear guard. Out of breath, having come off a night shift, just by some steep climbing had my claves and lungs taken fire. Was I a Thysis victim? I wandered.

Charlotte was first into the icy mountain pool, fed by a small cascading narrow waterfall, its sides slippery with moss and algae. Suddenly there came a shriek for help, one of the girls was having trouble swimming in the icy water. "I have a cramp in my leg" she shouted. A moment later the onlookers stood standing dumbstruck in horror, not moving my daughter didn't hesitate. She dived in head first, for seconds both heads were below the water. We were in panic, unable to help. All we could see was the boiling froth of water of the two people struggling under water. Suddenly just at it had suddenly begun both head popped out like champagne bottle corks. The girls didn't want the nun in charge to over react so the incident was kept hush-hush. Charlotte had been the hero for the weekend. At present she has Nico, who is husband and two karate boy's Tristan and the blond bomber Tyron. Charlotte that leader of her pack now has her great prized black belt, a fighter and a winner.

No Fear

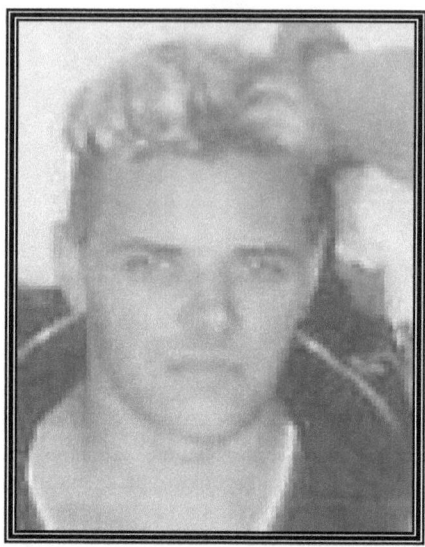

One thing my two sons had in common was no fear, no fear for speed. When it came to BMX racing whether it is off-road, through mud, sand, donga, sloot, ravine, desert, mountains, the bush, they went racing through it. It activated the adrenaline –pump, an exiting boost, a high for the body and spirit.

At the naughty age of runaway hormones, Quintin was no exception. He was the leader of the local BMX gang; "Rooikop" was second in charge and second fastest. As a gang they had a bad habit of racing through town, the ten of them, challenging the traffic from the opposite direction. This obviously caused consternation among the cars and would cause major traffic jam. The traffic cops were called out. This was part of the adrenaline rush for them. On hearing the distant whail of the fast approaching law, they would scatter in all directions, with a laugh and pat on the back. They would meet again at a designated place, where they would celebrate and tell how they got away.

Harmony mine at a place called Virginia had a well kept BMX racing track. Here Quintin and his friends joined the club. The dynamics of the racing, around the winding camel back track suited them and their need for speed. After a few months of racing Quintin and Patrick were both chosen to represent the Free State, a day of jubilation! On a certain day, a day of high drama, it was the day of reckoning, the championships for South African. Both boys were good at it and were super fit, legs muscles and calves highly developed. Tension on edge, their minds focused. The BMX track was well prepared, the crowds swarming over to look and strategize, those racers who didn't know the track, its sharp bends and pit-falls, the sudden falls. The day as set to be a bomb-shell, ready to explode, the tension at break point! Who would win and be the next BMX, SA champion?

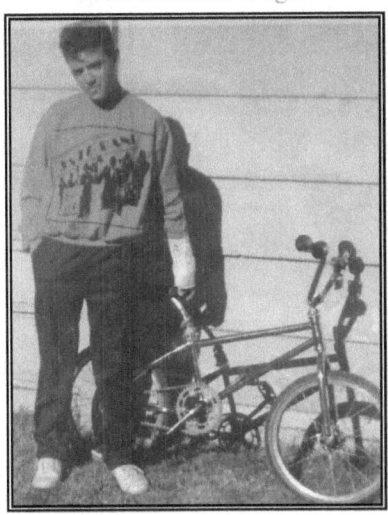

At the starting grid Quintin was ready for the race of his life. His multi-coloured safety helmet caused the salty sweat to pore down over his cheeks and eyes. In readiness for the start gun, all ten on the final line were ready to blast off, muscles tauty eyes focused ahead, the minds eye sweeping the track ahead, the winning post at the end. A split second of quietness before the report, its resounding crack, and the competitors were in a mad scramble, each one like a race horse at the July handi-cap to be in front. A great cheer went up, the commentators exited, speakers boom, heard.

Down the first straight they went at a steep 45 degree angle, and then a sharp bend and the hated high and very steep camel back. With out speed after the lower bend before, you would never make it's to the top, or make the race. Quintin knew this and was hoping those from afar would not, and this will be an advantage for him. At the first bend notorious for its collision a major pile up did occur. There riders with their mangled bikes and bodies lay. The others were still in the race. Over the camels back Quintin flew at high speed, pedals rotating madly, back hunched over the handles, eyes focused ahead. The commentator's exited voices came over the speakers. "Quintin Gird of the Free State team was a close second", it was a neck to neck finish, head to head. The crowds were on their feet, ecstatic. The two winners were like two rockets, passing the winning line a camera shot of a second between the two.

Who had won? Is Quintin our new South African Champion? Sadly for us he was voted a close second, but what a race! A race to be debated for years to come, Quintin was a champion in his own right anyway, the many medals and trophies line up in his room were the result of those mighty efforts. As a bonus for us, however Patrick our rising star came in first in the under five's, a new Junior SA champion, a smiling proud guy. Sadly a year later the mine due to finances closed down, the track and so did all the BMX riders aspirations. The type of determination did well and becoming a champion became a part of Quintin's "make-up" in his job and work situation. Traveling all over South Africa he gained experience, after leaving school as an Air-condition technician, he became a specialist in that field. From doing well in that car jammed city of Johannesburg, his wife Desa hated, they relocated to that scenic town called George, where this final story takes place.

The Beauty and the Beast

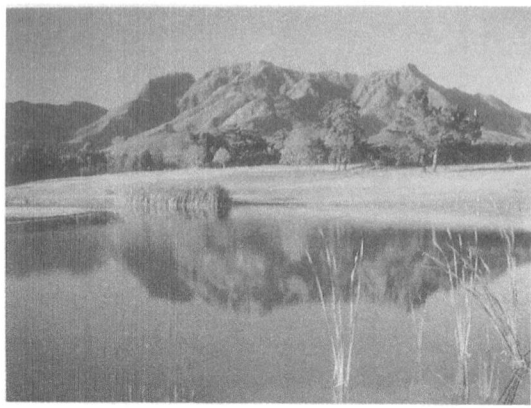

The town of George in the Western Cape is scenically most beautiful. Its surrounding is striking, astounding. On its one side flows the mighty turbulent Indian Ocean, its blue to green coloured water changing towards the deep blue-green haze far to the East. Its sound resounding among its rocky shore, on the west side stands majestically the Outeniqua range. Still and powerful, its peaks some times white capped. It also has a distant blue haze, a shimmering pulse, a life of its own.

In these peaceful surroundings a man doing his daily work nearly lost his life. He was to install a air-conditioner in a well to do Doctor's house, a old farm home in a rural area, while his helpers were off, loading the said air-conditioner this man went to inspect the installation place.

Enroot there he had to crawl through a dilapidated attic. The floor boards began cracking and splintering when ever he stepped a foot foreword. The lighting was dim. The room: unknown. He shivered. Suddenly the world around him exploded with the sound of rotting ceiling breaking under his weight. With a mighty splash he fell into a stagnant smelly, stinking pool of water. His muffled splattering cries for help were not heard. His body was covered with decaying weeds and green slime. He was caught in a giant spider web, a watery net of dark weeds. His efforts to escape became weaker. He was tiring quickly and nearly drowning: from his lips a quailing sound was cried.

His workers not hearing from him became alarmed and went to search for him. Strong arms and hands hoisted my son Quintin up, to safety. They had come just in time, helping hands. "God Sent". He won't forget that the Beast did not win that day. He is alive to tell all of his most lucky escape from drowning and the jaws of that dark Beast.

My son Quintin is stolen 1980

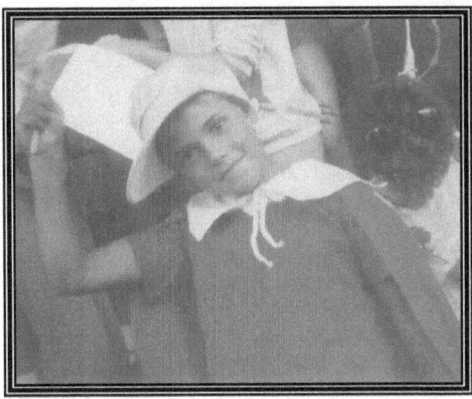

A number of decisions lead to my son being stolen, the modern term used in the media would be "hi – Jacked", or "kidnapped". Fortunately in this case there was no ransom demand only an apology, an apology so poor in motivation it would make you puke in disgust.

The decision I refer to were the deciding of where to go to for our annual leave, shortly due. To the sea or an inland holiday, would this year be different? I mused through the many brochures advertising the many inland resorts to go to. Would it be the challenge of boating over the murky brown waters of the great expanse of inland waters, the Vaal dam, or canoeing, speed boating, sailing along the willow tree-lined the Vaal River. Fishing? No, I wasn't a fisherman to save my life as it were, the story goes that the modern fisherman doesn't fish but "looks into the bottle deeply", they call it "looking for answers or solitude there in" Married to a bottle! Bird watching, seeing those high flying and shrill call of the fish eagle, in search of fish food? Hiking routs, the Vredefort dome where there the evidence of a outer space meteor strike of many years ago, its crater a hiking trail, or the San bushman paintings. Abseiling from the sand stone abutments, rock climbing. The Eastern Free State well known to me with its familiar changing topography from flat to hilly to the sudden stark rugged sand stone cliffs, the majestic Malutis or the winding "dragon mountain" in a way it looked as if they were keeping a watchful eye over its neighbor, the grassy flat lands, inferior to "their majesty" below them.

Other holiday resorts were closer to home, the well known Golden Gate Reserve and all its attractions there. The Caledon River which rises in the Berg just described, its caves, sloping sides, its lairs hidden, hideaways, ramparts, evidence of battle fields long gone.

In conclusion with Martie and the children it was anonymously decided to go seawards, there was no other choice, they were adamant. It was like a year to year ritual. After loading the new Ford Fairlain V-8 with what we needed we were on our way, following the rout form Welkom, East wards, over the great Van Reenen Pass through the Natal midlands, eventually to the shores of the famous Zululand. We arrived before day light, a stiff breeze blowing. The early morning sun was creeping up over the horizon's rim, a dull ball of flame, its heat would be felt later. The row upon row of waves coming and going pounded the coast line, the spray seen, the booming sound heard from a mile off, we felt glad to be there. Relaxing after the long night drive, sitting in the car you searched the oceans waters expanse and saw no end to it, a mass too big to imagine. The misty haze started turning from a dark purple to a light blue as the suns warmth and rays became brighter.

The children were soon playing excitedly, passing the ball to each other or running head long into the waves. Martie had her picnic basket out and before long we were having our brunch of bore wors, boiled eggs, fresh home made bread and sweet steaming coffee. We were really having a good time, the modern teenage term was "chilling out" forgotten were our problems and worries but unknown to us by the end of that day we would be more than worried, a shocking incident would rear its ugly head.

By mid-day the crowds had accumulated to a few hundred in number, holiday makers, bathers, a great assembly of humanity, a coming and going of activity, as if it was a live dynamo in action, having a life of its own. We felt the energy of the sun its rays burning us to a dark brown bronze. This was the life! Towards mid afternoon Martie came to me, a worried look on her face, Quintin was missing. That in itself was not unusual, all children get lost at one time or another, but were quickly found.

Holding a tense family meeting we discussed where we had searched and to whom did we ask for help, the SAP, No, the life savers, No, our car, No, the boating area, No, to all my questions asked the answer was negative. Quintin had vanished into thin air, as it were. Our search widened futher away to the dense bushy area, where the many campers were. Through the thick vegetation we saw a family breaking camp, the sun was setting and they were homeward bound.

Martie now in a frenzy of worry went to enquire. Next to an old beat up Fiat stood a middle aged slovenly woman supervising, her families departure. Standing close to the vehicle Martie saw a familiar figure sitting hunched up on the back seat. It was Quintin! Pushing the hag out of the way, she yanked the door open and shouted, "Quintin, What are you doing here? We are all worried about you, why are you here?" She pulled him out, giving him a mother's hug of relief. With angry blazing eyes she whirled on to the child abductor and said, "Why have you stolen my son? It is against the law to steal children, kidnappers can go to jail for a long time."
Caught out in her dirty act the women answered in accented English, "I lost my son years ago, this lovely boy looks like him, and we were now departing to our home in Rio, South America." She sobbed, head bowed in shame. Martie and I too shocked to answer stood rooted to the ground, we would have lost Quintin forever, and even the thought of that day haunts us. What if it really did happen? A family tragedy was averted.

We told the perpetrator to get going fast out of South Africa, or we would call the police. We were to glad to have out son back to worry about making a case. Martie's rage subsided, relenting being a loving mother herself we turned and left the depressing scene. It was time to move on. We packed the fairlaine and drove southwards to Margate; the Margate Gird's were waiting for us.

Unsteady

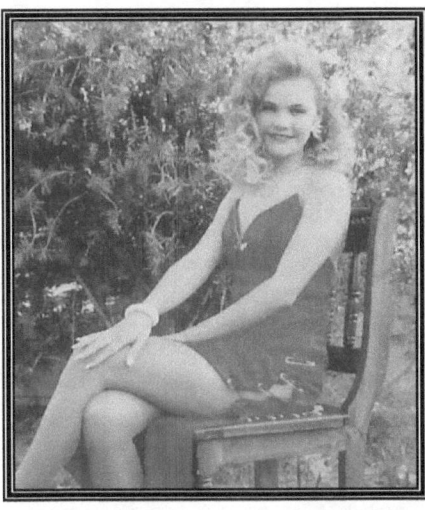

There are many things Angelique did. She was and is the most beautiful girl in the world – and uses this power and gift to full advantage. Combining with her striking femininity is her loving nature. All who meet her, especially those who work closely with her on a daily basis, her work colleagues and more importantly her family? I as her Dad should know, from her earliest age I took her to pre-school on the handle bars of the bike in rain or strong winds without fail.

As mentioned she was a doer not a sitter. What she did, she did with meaning and determination. To prove my point when doing ballet, she was the star of the class, winning many trophies. Her suppleness, and grace on the floor won the day. Her whole family did Karate; she joined us and went on to obtaining her orange belt. She was through the ballet training, so supple that her kicks in the air were the best. On the athletic field her potential was great.

She trained as a Hotel manager to start off in that career. You have to start at the bottom, and that was waitressing in the Log Hotel in Knysna. Her future look rosy, I am not quite sure how her present boss found her and her talent, but it was in the same vein, touching people. This was done through a better pay offer. In a few years she became manager to this firm, a dynamic sales women and leader though example. Her crowning moment was the birth of a most beautiful gift from heaven, a baby girl called Veronique. Safry is her devoted husband.

With all these attributes she was and is unsteady, unsteady not as on her feet, but on a bicycle. From an early age her sister Lillian lifted her on her bike to school. The many bikes I bought her were to no avail, she either fell, losing her balance, went over an unfortunate cat, now dead. She was the target of all types of hounds and dogs. The biggest and most viscous attacked her and her pink bike, black or what ever colour I bought her. Even when doing matric a huge rodweiler went for her. Why? Nobody knows. Trying to get her car license hopefully won't be a problem. Let's hope there is no unsteadiness behind the cars steering wheel and won't bring other cars to attack her! Hopefully when she does get her license she wont go over any cats or dogs herself.

Determination

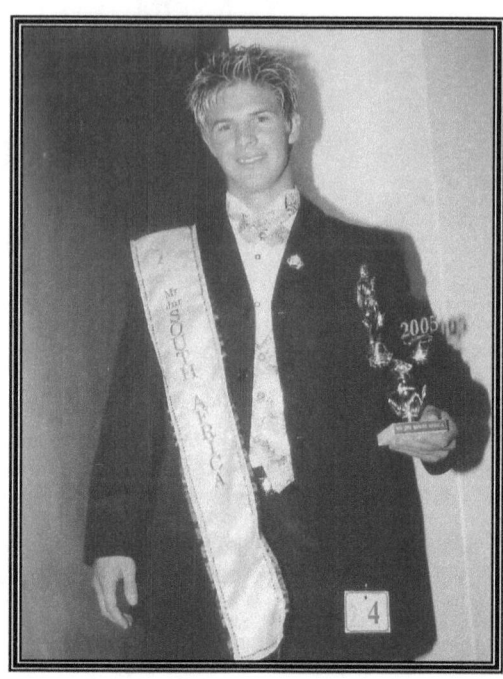

Patrick Walter Gird is different to the rest of my children. The word to be used was fearless. He could climb the highest tree where ever it was, in a park in Johannesburg or at home. He had no phobia over heights. A normal brick made building, its wall in particular was a challenge. One day to my horror I found him climbing straight up ABSA Bank's walls. At 10m, I called him down in a gentle tone of voice as not to scare him or that he may panic at my urgent call. He was only three years old. Down he came at the cheering of a crowd just gathered to watch the excitement.

At home on calling him he would be found on top of the house roof, playing with his toys. He would either shin up quickly the gutters pipe or up the brick wall by finger power as mountain climbers do on the mighty Alps. The most disturbing thing was when called to dinner or homework, off the roof he would jump. Landing on his two feet expertly, later this would be detrimental to his feet bones, a crumbling action would occur.

His elder brother Quintin showed him the finer points of BMX riding and racing. This was a sport this boy loved. It had all the ingredients to foster his determined adventurous indomitable fighting spirit. All over S.A. they traveled for competitions. At the age of 5 this boy became a S.A.-BMX champion. Unfortunately their BMX racing track sponsored by a local mine was stopped. The track today is covered with grass and bush, a reminder of what was and what could have been, a breeding ground for future champions?

Through and up to the age of 13, he played school sport at Welkom PREP, but did not excel at cricket, rugby or swimming. He was very interested in Karate and would always be in a rough and tumble, a shirt torn or a bleeding lip would come as a result. His mother was not pleased. The age of 14, I took him to the local TAE KWON DO a self defense club. That first session was a disaster. While doing mock fighting he received a vicious high kick to the ear. Crying with impotent rage he wanted to go home and give up. The result was the opposite in effect. Two years later, after grading to blue belt and winning many championships he was chosen to be included in the Springbok team to compete nationally for S.A.

He did exceptionally well in London, England, at Johannesburg airport on his return he was given a heroes Welkom. Having reached the top of that sport, the challenge met, he had his site on other fields of endeavors, to quicken that indomitable spirit of him.

He chose a most unlikely past time, one in which I didn't have much faith in, modeling. Would he succeed this time? Doing the complete opposite, to what he was used to doing in a contact sport.

A good friend of his, Richard introduced him to the glamour world. From the age of 14 to 18 this boy climbed the ladder of success. His athletic build, poise and grace on stage, his elegant attire won him the day. His mother, Martie was his back-stop and without that he would mot have made it to the top, one reason being that Martie was an ex-modeling champion herself knowing the finer details, what to wear and when; required discipline.

At his modeling school he practiced hard on the ramp, doing all the stopping and turning at the right time. After winning the Mr. Welkom Square, he went on competing in the different provinces, eventually winning the cover title of Mr. Junior Free State.

He was now eligible to compete for the S.A. title.

At a glittering gala event in Benoni he became Mr. Junior South Africa, a proud young man, someone his mother and father were especially proud of.

His year of reign was most exciting, visiting old age homes and children's hospitals through out South Africa.

That determined boy, now a man, is and will always be my son, the fearless one, the need for speed one, the determined one, apart of my Autobiography, a part of the future.

To date he has won Mr. King of the Universe

Vista

1992

Klein grootman

nnie Hennop

...ETSRY is vir kinders
...s ongewoon nie, maar
...a op vyfjarige ouderdom

oud was, begin BMX ry.
Onlangs het hy aan die SA
kampioenskappe in Pieter-
maritzburg deelgeneem en
'n goue- en 'n silwer me-
dalje verower.

Sy broer Quintin (16)
is ook 'n ervare BMX-jaer.
Hy was Patrick se rolmo-
del en het selfs sy klein-
boet se fiets gebou.

Volgens sy ma was Pa-
trick saam toe Quintin een
dag aan 'n wedren deelge-
neem het. Daarna het hy
op 'n fiets geklim en begin
ry.

Hy kon ook die die
baan met hindernisse vol-
tooi, sonder enige onder-
steuning van sy pa. Ge-
woonlik moet die klein-
tjies se pa's hulle oor 'n
paar van die hindernisse
help.

Volgens sy ouers is Pa-
trick dol oor fietsry. "In
die oggend moet my man
met die motorfiets agter
Patrick aan ry na sy speel-
groep toe. Patrick dring
eenvoudig daarop aan om
met sy fiets na die speel-
groep te ry.

"Ons moet net keer, as
die hek oop is, wil hy net
strate toe met sy fiets. Hy
is toegewyd oor die sport
en is 'n vasberade jaer," sê
sy ma.

Patrick, wat tans in die
beginner-afdeling ry, sal
eers op agtjarige ouder-
dom 'n kans kry om vir
provinsiale en nasionale
titels te jaag — en wie
...et, dalk is hy die volgende SA kampioen.

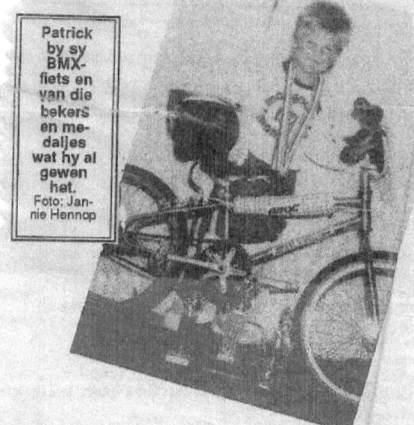

Patrick
by sy
BMX-
fiets en
van die
bekers
en me-
daljes
wat hy al
gewen
het.
Foto: Jan-
nie Hennop

al aan professionele
BMX-kampioenskappe
deel te neem, is nie elke
kind beskore nie.
    Klein Patrick Gird van
Welkom het reeds verlede
jaar, toe hy maar vier ja

Hy het reeds n sy kort
sportloopbaan tintalle bekers en medalje gewen.
Hy het ry ook sof in an-
der klein Vrystertjies se
...

The Angry Sea

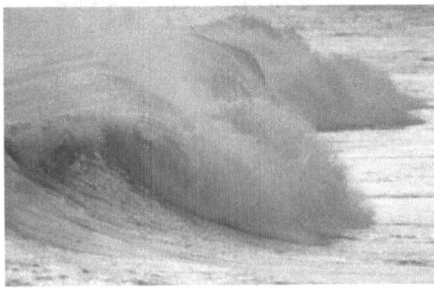

Andries, my daughter Charlotte's in law, worked on the gold mines in the Free State, Welkom. Here more that a million people have made their homes. This town has a high level of infrastructure supporting it. The new name for the Gold fields is Lejweleputswa, meaning grey stones. Welkom is now called Mathjabeng, its economy is build around the mining of gold and agriculture.

Deep in the bowels of the earth sat Andries in one of these mines, he was in deep thought and dejected. He wasn't happy with his present work environment, period. By nature he was an out door person, his favourite past time was fishing at the local dams or rivers. In his minds eye he could see the great Indian Ocean, the refreshing wet breeze on his cheek, the waves parting as he drove his high powered twin turbo speed boat through those frothing waves. How ever his reverie was interrupted by the coming of the noisy approach of the underground local pulling its full eight ton hoppers. The iron wheels were making a screaming sound as they came around the tunnel bend. The regulatory siren was wailing its warning, the loco battery operated, the mine being a fiery mine so that a spark would not ignite and cause a explosion, had its strong head light on, the light stabbing and lighting up the pitch darkness ahead.

At the back of this train sat the Loco guards man to assist if a sudden derailment would occur and the help when the tonnage was tipped at the main tips. Andries now sat in his office to avoid the dust as the "entourage" went past. The area was well wetted down but due to the spillage of the over loaded hoppers the dust became intolerable. It brought with if unwanted Thysis. He had on the breathing mask, but unfortunately he already had thysis, first grade. He knew what it meant, the bearer there of would having a incurable lung disease, this meant that the lungs became so clogged up with microscopic particles of dust that it became as it were a non porous paper bag opening and shutting with no purpose to the human body. Thus the stricken person would die of asphyxiation, a terrible slow death.

Coming back to his life long dream of relocating to the sea, he was more determined to go, but how? He stifled a chocking cough, tears streaming from him red eyes, his hatred of his circumstances growing day by day. However fate took a hand. On arriving back at home he was puzzled to find an official letter from the mine pension board, with a wide grin he called Iris his wife, the letter state that he was qualified to leave on his present age and time historically worked on the mines. The man and wife pair agreed that their health was more important than money; they would full fill that life dream and live at the sea. With a lump sum pay out, Andries bought a sea going boat, V-6 car to pull it and off they went.

At a coastal resort called Hibberdene they settled down, my daughter Charlotte, Nico her husband and small boy Tristan joined them there. Their idea was to do business by fishing and holiday makers paying for deep sea trips. Nico and his dad studied for their skipper's licenses and passed with flying colours, they could now do legitimate business. Martie, Patrick and I decided to go on holiday and pay them a friendly visit. The welcomed us with open arms. By this time the two Bouwers were good at reading the weather, so as to decide whether or not to go boating. I was invited to go with the next day; I was over joyed, as I had never gone deep sea fishing before.

The weather was fine the next morning, the tractor towards the boat to the pier on the river; here the boats would be sent off to the sea after offloading the boat on to the river water, the boat now floating, we clambered on, Nico, Andries and I were on our way. Soon the twin turbo engines were started, its high pitched wine becoming a shriek. The front of the boat lifted, we were moving forward at high speed, cutting the smooth water like a knife through soft butter. To get to the ocean from the river side required a skippers skill because facing you were those high waves rushing ferociously at you, Nico at the helm, powered the boat though each wave expertly, the waves met with a thud of the underside, the spray covering us. Suddenly we were out in the open, the sea beaconing us, as it were.

The fish finder, an ingenious method by means of a computer warned us of fish under us. The engines were stopped, the fishing rods taken out and also the "pad kos "thick home made sandwiches, dripping with honey, after an hour we called it a day, there were no bites. Starting the twin powered, we ploughed on, a plume of white spray on either side of the boat. Interesting we saw a big whale and its calf. We headed eastwards to no avail, no fish in sight. The day had started with a wonderful calm, the sea a turquoise blue, with no grey threatening clouds to be seen, without warning those clouds not seen before now appeared ominously, and were now approaching us at great speed from the dark east. The sea turned a dark grey, becoming choppy and unpleasant in a matter of minutes the weather had changed for the worse; it became a boiling mass of danger to us. Out of now where a huge "tsunami type" of wave rushed on to us, covering the boat in seconds. We were drenched to the bone. We nearly capsized. Andries shouted "ons moet nou huis toe gaan, hier gaan ons vrek" meaning we had better turn back home ward as soon as possible. Luckily the boat had all the latest navigational equipment, with Nico at the helm, who knew what to do, he was now in charge, a man of few words with a black belt in karate, and we were bumping on a roller coaster as it were. The sea was in a bad mood, the wind velocity increased to a howl, rising to a crescendo. I was terrified mainly because of the dangerous circumstances and not knowing where the coast was or what direction we were taking. The visibility was null, darkness pervading us.

Suddenly Andries shouted that he could make out the shore, on closer inspection we were happy to see the sands of Hibberdene. Motoring faster to get past the roaring waves, Nico landed the boat directly on to the soft sand, with a thump the boat hit the beach sliding up the for about ten meters. We were safe! Andries and Nico were in their element, but I was not, I don't think I will venture quickly on to the sea again. May be I am a coward, but rather be a live one, than a dead one!

The Free State, Welkom 1990

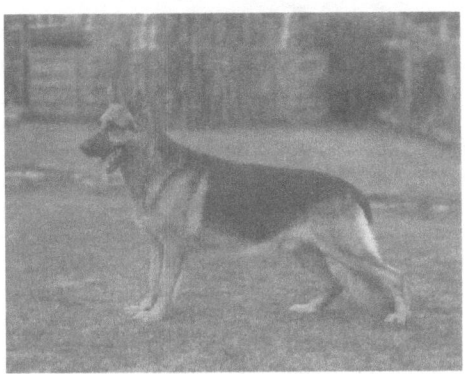

Our Dog Dudie

The gold Mine used to spoil its workers by allowing them cheap, affordable housing. They were either made of asbestos or back face brick. We lived in an asbestos house that was designed to last for 10 years, so we did not take the offer by the company and buy one, hoping to purchase a brick one, we moved to a suburb called Flamingo Park.

This home-stead's been a vast improvement, spacious room and well placed gardens with fruit trees. This area was set aside by the company mainly for its officials. That was an advantage, but also a disadvantage. Adjacent to all these "well-to-do" families was a giant open field. This was criss-crossed by mine commuters. The either worked at a nearby shaft or were from a undesirable element from the black town ship Thabong. These "fly-by-nights were past masters at home theft.

The more successfully the broke in with out stoppage, the bolder they became. Mostly they come by stealth and not by force. Friends of ours were watching intently at soccer one night and on going to bed found no furniture left. Stealing wasn't only during the night, your washing on the line if not watched, it went missing before you got back from town. Garden appliances were in the same category, a thief's game. The Glintenkamp family of ours, daughter Linda, came running to us, out of breath, to tell us that their house had been burgled. Now traumatized rushed to their house to find the place in a mess. The thieves had gotten away with radios, televisions, money, blankets and food. Winton in a wild rage drove off in search of the perpetrators. He had a Ford Passat motor car, which we used to call "Pas gekoop en sat gery" he wasn't amused by the joke.

The insurance did pay out, but it became alarmingly unsafe. Angelique having had her bike stolen, borrowed one of the Glintenkamp's children bike to get go school. At the convent the sister-nun could only watch helplessly as a thief rode away with it, just before she was going to lockup the bicycle shed.

Another family in Welkom was busy moving to Rustenburg. They were well organized, and were ready for the removal lorry to come. The furniture was stacked on the side-walk to be loaded. As planned a red lorry came along and loaded everything up. With smiles and promising to see them in Rustenburg the went off- an hour later another red removal lorry came, after much confusion and swearing it was ascertained that the first one had "hi-jacked" their belongings!

A friend of ours across the road from us had a house with a high fence. Beside that he had a huge black Rodweiler dog as protection. No one went hear there because when this beast jumped up and down you could see his huge head, fangs and slime running down his jaws ready to bit your head off. The school children would throw stones at him, laugh and run away. The owner Loius was proud to boast that no one would dear to steal from him. He was proved to be wrong. Through an ingenious plan, the crooks did get in. In his safe was stacks of cash, the bar was well stocked with all the best and expensive liquor. The fridge was full of meat and delicacies. After the dirty deed was done we pieced the story together like a jig-saw puzzle. The perpetrators having their eye on the house for a long time lurked the "black lion" to the front gate. They did this by bringing temptation, a bitch on heat. This fierce dog came out of the yard like a lamb to the slaughter, meekly, following the bitch into an enclosed bakkie. His member extended like a large red carrot. They were quickly shut up. The door tightly closed the rodweilers duty to his master now forgotten. The servant girl was conveniently away for the weekend. Louis and his family were visiting friends. The thieves raided the house. Everything of value was taken. The house was ransacked. The pedigree rodweiler was never seen again. Rumors going around said, that the beast was now used for a super stud. The thieves would make more money from the off springs. The family was disgusted, and later moved to a safer area.

In this atmosphere and tension Martie decide to shop around for good and well bread German shepherd dog. Seeing an advertisement in the local news paper we contacted the breeders at a placed called Maselspoort near Bloemfontein. We drove there to the said breeder's farm and purchased two magnificently bred, above mentioned dogs. Loading them up, with their papers to prove family history we drove back to Welkom. We named them Dudie and Moncherie. They were already trained and a year old with no puppies. They were smaller in statue than the normal Alsations. Their back hair was covered in a shining reddish sheen, the male bigger that his female counter part, both strong agile, well muscled and full of life. Their heads gave a radiance of quality, clean cut and nobility. The muzzles long and strong, forehead slightly arched and not domed or rounded. The ears pointed to the front and open. Their teeth still young, sharp and strong, their eyes oval in shape similar to those wolves in the wild, showing keenness and intelligence. Their long powerful legs characteristic of the breed, they had all the attributes of the German shepherd, good character, quiet confidence, always willing to serve their master, never tired. Our two did have bad habits, one was they hated poodles. On one occasion, one had inadvertently strolled into our yard from no reason. The front gate being open, this unlucky white poodle was found under a bush in the corner of the yard bitten to death. I won't describe what he looked like, a bloody mess.

It was safe to say, around that area most homesteads were broken into, but ours was untouched up to this day. The combination of both dogs on patrol, up and down the fence was too dawn ting for any thief to try and steal off the premises. They became legendary. A basic illness some get is arthritis. Dudie was no exception; her back was affected the most and in her old age was bed ridden, lying sill inactive, and a sorry sight. I was forced to put her out. With tears streaming down my face I made the grave.
She was our first, we won't forget.

Martie and the Indian Ocean 1990

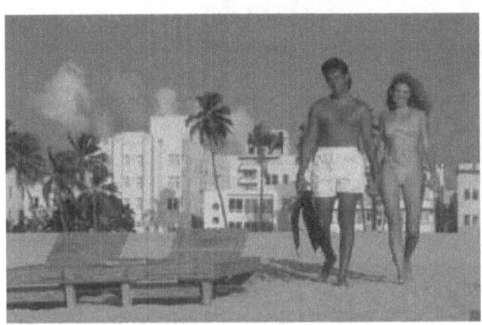

No one wants to die, whether by drowning, thirst, fire, Aids, or body cells mutilating such as having that dreaded disease called cancer.

But if any of us have had a near death experience then our whole out look on life changes for ever. What happens? We are forced to come out of that pleasure zone. I my case, I can attest to two near death experiences, the first being a terrible and horrific mine accident, and presently the on going battle against lymph gland cancer. Why, I am being so melodramatic about death is that my wife, Martie, also had a harrowing near death experience at the hands of the Indian Ocean.

Being on our annual leave and driving from the "Big sky country", the Free State, we as a family were looking forward to our rest at the sea. We would be getting together with the Margate Girds, a happy reunion. In our excitement to get there we would bet who would see the sea first, and who would get into the water first! The next day on getting up I would be the first to sit and stare out onto the misty sea. Many thoughts would go through my mind. It felt good to have the refreshing and salty sea breeze on my face. Watching the waves they would come in wave after wave, rolling on high of 2 meters, then stop for a fraction, the drop thunderous on to the sea sand. This continues onslaught would also be directed to the nearly rocks, only the variety, velocity and speed would chop and change. On top of this receding water is always a white froth. The Basotho whom I grew up with referred it as Bagoa, or whites, meaning that we came by sea and should go back the way we Europeans came.

This sea could be tranquil at times, at other times moody and unpredictable, come times even cruel. Some violent, unforgiving like us humans. This deadly coast, especially along the wild coast, and the Port Elizabeth are, a great danger to man and ships, their graves and wrecks below the sea. This great expanse of ocean had a life of its own. It has a pulling effort on us, a gigantic magnetism soothing for the soul. It also had a medic nary value, a bowel cleansing action when drunk! On the beach would be those highly muscled life savers. They would have exercised by swimming a mile, jogging 10 km. They were to save lives of those inexperienced swimmers. The terrain of unseen underwater currents and the vicious back wash was well known to them. They were ready for the day. The sun would come up in the East, the dark gray blue changing to a brighter blue and in the distance a haze green.

As this was happening in nature, the holiday comers were descending on to the beach, in all shapes and sizes. The day began to get stifling hot, the crowds flocked into the refreshing coolness of the sea. Martie and I were holding hands, as usual as a gesture of love and security. The children were playing happily at the waters edge, they were safe. Martie let go of my hand for a moment to go floating or body surfing. Suddenly an underwater current gave a jerk, she cried out. My hand out stretched. With in a few seconds she was swept out to sea, the rocks looming to the left. Martie being a good swimmer had her fist held high in a ball, a universal sigh of distress.

In panic not being able to help, not being a good swimmer, I made as quickly as I could to look for any life saver to help. None could be seen. Sobbing with frustration I arrive at there radio center, banging on the door, no one. Turning around in desperation, stumbling back none were seen. In my misery a voice came to me, in my depressed state saying, "Your wife is now safe, we have rescued her just in time." The life savers had done their work well! I found her sitting dejectedly crying, crying for being safe and shocked at the recent harrowing near death experience. Up to this day she is angry at me for abandoning her and not rescuing her, but also understands the forces of the sea, loving to be there, but knowing its power.

Chapter 5

Cancer: Unknown forces strike!

Chapter 5 Cancer: Unknown forces strike!

1. Cancer: The emotional break down

The shock!

My mother died after along sickbed, after breaking both hip joints one after the other. Being over the age of 88 the pain and shock was too much, she died in the arms of Mike and Janis, having had extreme support from the priest. After the funeral the shock came to me. A great pain in the chest, could it be a heart attack? No, not according to the Dr Bardenhorst, it was an angina attack, tension of the muscles around the heart which was giving the pain. On further examination he saw a swelling on the left side of my neck and a giant swelling on the left side of the abdomen. I was a worried man. After the specialist had seen me, a Biopsy was done.

It was found to be malignant cancer of the lymph glands. Denial by me! The hour of death had arrived. The shock was too much, but I held on to sanity. Why me? I could not be sick. I am a healthy man. I led a healthy life style, eating the correct foods, exercising, walking a lot with regular weight training, all for nothing?

OBVIOUSLY it was an outside attack beyond my control!

The enemy had broken through. The last year or two, I felt at times drained, without energy and very tired. I felt vulnerable, was it the enemy who had slipped in, then I felt angry. Silent recrimination, frustration, helplessness were all the feelings going through my mind. I was infected the cancer was eating me alive. Could this feel worse that Aids? Is this how they feel, I have my deepest sympathy for them now. Only a person with a life threatening disease would know what a person is going through. Being told you have malignant cancer is a shock. After the denial stage, what is going to be done about it?

The emotions pouring through one comes like a stormy whirlwind, devastating everything in its path. The uncertainty, the not knowing what is ahead, the gloom of the future, is it about living your last in pain, or are you going to turn the boat around?

On hearing the news the cancer association sister sent a trained sister to comfort me and give me advice. I refused to be given any solace as I believed there was basically nothing wrong with me. I told her over the phone I was not sick and did not want hear her or see her.

How could I be sick today but perfectly healthy yesterday, training with weights and went for long walks and all? I was arrogant; my body was not made for any diseases. I would fight it all the way; information was what I needed to fight this unknown intruder.

Planning thoughts

I am fighting for my life, against an enemy unknown and determined to take my life.
I am not going to allow it to happen, I am not meant to be sickly and die before my time.

How am I going to plan this counter attack?
By using the information at my disposal I am going to plan my day to day walking and talking on a schedule.

From the uncertainty we move to the certainty.

- ❖ How do we do this?
- ❖ Find out what is going on.
- ❖ What type of cancer have I got?
- ❖ For information go to the nearest library and read up all relevant information on your type of cancer.
- ❖ Ask your Doctor and Oncologist.
- ❖ Join the Cancer Association COPING groups; they support you mentally and physically.

2. At the Oncologist - Dr Lion Cachet

Being a women doctor with many years of extensive experience she was very knowledgeable and understanding. Looking at the CAT scan she explained in detail what the scan meant, because to us lay men it was not unintelligible. She showed the CAT scan to Martie, Lillian and I where the huge tumor was and where the other swollen glands on the neck:

1. We saw the tumor sitting just below the left abdomen muscle, as big as a rat. To extract it would do no good because there were far too many and extracting one would have no purpose.
2. Huge clusters of glands like grapes were hanging around the swollen neck to the left and right sides.
3. The chest area was infected but not as badly as the rest.
4. The liver was enlarged and so was the spleen infected.
5. The heart was normal.
6. The lungs, intestines, lower glands and testicles were fine, so was the prostrate.

The Oncologist was feeling abnormal glands from the neck down. She was worried about the enlarged tumor in the abdomen. She worked out my forth coming 8 chemo therapy strengths and chemical dosage to my weight, age and general health noted, I would have to see her at least once a month to monitor the progress, the effects of the chemo, positive and negative sides. She was quite sure that the cancer had reached the blood, which in such cases was normal. I had to get a bone marrow graft to ascertain whether the cancer had reached the blood or not.

The bone marrow extraction was done, but painfully. A bone was extracted with a sample of marrow. This was put in a small bottle and shown to me. The specimens were sent to Bloemfontein for testing at the lab. The next night at 5 pm the Oncologist phoned. The news was fantastic, the cancer had not reached the blood, and she regarded it as a stage when the cancer could be stopped in its unholy march, just in time.

The eight Chemo sessions taking place from
5/09/2005 to 04/04/2006

To tell about them is not a pleasant task. The first being the worst, the reason being is by not being prepared, for what was to happen to me. The worst experience was the intestine blockage. To have a swollen tummy is not a joke, castor oil, endocots, DPO depositories had no effect. My anus was like a swollen ball, unable to blow down and deflate, it was painful. After 5 days nature took over and normality came back. It taught me a great lesson, take laxative before the chemo!

The other side effects were:

- ❖ Headaches
- ❖ Nausea
- ❖ Throwing up
- ❖ Bad tempers
- ❖ Emotional
- ❖ Pins and needles in the feet
- ❖ Cramps in the legs
- ❖ Dizziness
- ❖ Hot and cold flushes
- ❖ Tiredness during the day (a short nap usually helped)

After 7 months of chemo discomfort I went to the doctor again with a review scan. The result were beyond any joy, the cancer, the enemy to my body was gone. With tears of happiness she explained by comparing the first scan to the newest one, how the tumor had shrunk to the size of a small pebble. Hopefully not malignant, the clusters of grape like swollen glands were gone.

On her thorough body exam she corroborated the findings of the scan report, I was clean.
She exclaimed that I was one of the lucky ones, the others were not so lucky. She was well pleased. One last objective would be to go to Johannesburg for a final scan. Any malignant cells would be found on this new machine from the United States. But at this stage the Medical aid will only pay for this examination if there I showed no progress in the treatment had received.

3. What to do, via information?

Further Cancer information at the Library
To find books on the subject would bring light to this darkness. I checked the following books before going to the Oncologist.

What do the Medical books say about cancer?
What is cancer?
There are 200 forms of cancer. The cells in the body go out of control. They are divided into two groups:

* ❖ *Group 1: cells in organs such as in the lungs and breasts*
* ❖ *Group 2: this type of cancer goes from the connective of the muscles, bones, and blood, lymphoma-lymph glands, the digestive system, and intestines.*

Definition in Webster English Dictionary:
It is a malignant growth, tending to metastasizes and multiply destructively in the body.

Definition in Medical and Health Encyclopedia:
A disease characterized by abnormal and unpredictable growth of cells, they invade normal healthy tissues which they destroy.

Effects of the destruction of the cells are:
* ❖ *Pain*
* ❖ *Nerve damage*
* ❖ *Blood vessel infected*
* ❖ *Hemorrhaging*
* ❖ *Lung defunct ions*
* ❖ *Kidney failure*
* ❖ *Artery blockage and abnormalities*
* ❖ *Bladder problems*

It affects the following:
Destroying tissues as it grows as it multiplies in size and destroying all before it. The breasts, digestive system, genitals, the unitary system, the flow and spread in the blood or the lymphatic glands through out the body. The glands act as barriers to infection. Once infected themselves by cancerous cells they self multiply and become larger and larger, if not stopped a person could become paralyzed which will lead to a slow death.

The exact cause of cancer is not known, but we do know that cancer cells are not normal cells. Some direct causes we do know are cancer of the lip is through pipe smoking. Cancer of the lungs is through cigarette smoking chemicals. Skin cancer is through rays of the sun. The female cur vex, sex hormones affecting breast and genital cancer. The incorrect use of the X-ray machinery can cause cancer.

Methods of Diagnosis: Biopsy:
What is a biopsy?
It is the removal of a cancerous cell by means of surgery. This cancerous cell is tested by chemicals in a lab or viewed under a microscope.

What are the usual signs of cancer?
In the blood it manifest itself causing anemia, fatigue, swelling of the lymph glands, pain, loss of weight, short of breath and abnormal tiredness after exercise, loss of strength and loss of muscle tissue.

What are the different forms of treatment found?
1. The removal of the cancerous growth.
2. Treatment by radium
3. Chemo therapy drug management and control.
4. Radio activity treatment, combined with radio active therapy.
5. Isotopes.
6. Hormonal therapy.

What is Hodgkin's disease?
Involves the lymph gland and their enlargement and infection, it usually spreads from neck on either side. It can spread to the liver enlarging it, the spleen, bone marrow, spine or vertebrae, paralysis the lower body.

Type of Hodgkin's disease:
The slow and the fast, the slow can be controlled better, the fast more difficult. The Oncologist decides how and when and what therapy to give.

Symptoms:
❖ Loss of weight
❖ Ill health
❖ The body wasting away
❖ Enlarged glands, with painful swelling
❖ Chest pains
❖ Coughing, pressure on the trachea
❖ Difficulty in swallowing
❖ Breathing difficulty and very painful
Different therapies:
1. Radiation
2. Chemo
3. Removal

4. Wally's thoughts on how to win!

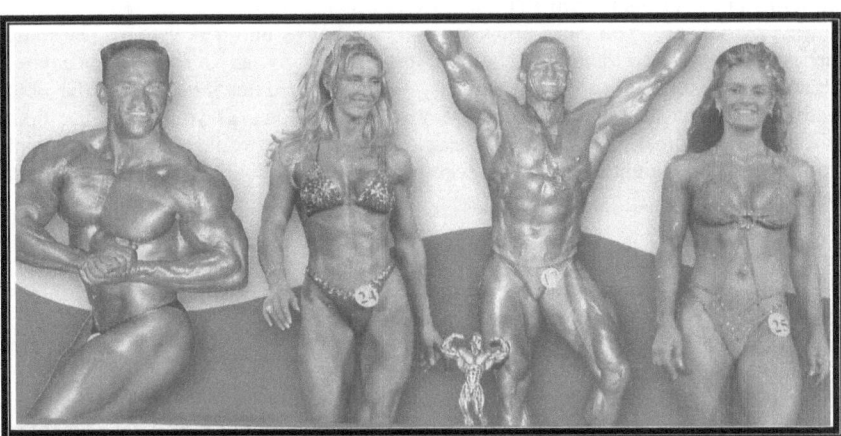

Take action by taking one day at a time

My daily schedule

Plan the day ahead. It's a mental exercise. It's an exercise of the will power. Being mental means you are able to see in the minds eye what you are going to do, not for the next week, month, or year but for that one day only. There is no place for the negative, drive it out now. Goal's, I set must be attainable for example if I can't get up at 6 am then be a little flexible and make it later, but still stick to the daily plan, step by step, piece by piece that mountain is going to move and is now moving away.

What is in store for the day? Make it exiting. Do it yourself instead of other people fetching your coffee, making it yourself, it is about fulfilling your objective. Sitting is being inactive; inactivity means regressing, going backwards, which according to my schedule I put up, is not allowed.

Back to basics; make that porridge yourself in the mornings. Feed the dog, cats and birds, keep moving. I am paranoiac about it, don't lying down and feel sorry for yourself, be happy you are alive and not dying. The reason why I feel like this is the emotional experience I went through after the horrific mine accident. I saw many people give up. The pain and shock they are going through is just too much. They stop eating, drinking, refuse to listen to the Doctor and Nurses orders. They feel self pity, depressed and by refusing medication their life expectancy is shortened.

While I lay in ICU a man of 50 had a hip replacement, but through pain and shock and refusing to eat or drink, to my horror on the 1999/01/01he died. There are many cases of cancer patients where they succumbed to pain and misery, they got worse, the chemo being too much, and they passed away unnecessarily with out any real resistance. Obviously if the cancer has progressed too far and too quickly, or not stopped in time, you are not dead until God say so. Miracles still

From Darkness to light

happen, I am one. Being positive keeps me alive, a living faith burning, prayers continuously going up to heaven what ever the thoughts or emotions.

What is planned for the rest of the day? A walk in the park or do a few sit-ups, a short visit to the gym in town or your home gym. Those muscles can't be allowed to slacked or become soft, wither away, or deflate. You can't allow yourself to change into a skeleton. The muscles is what carries you, so to feed them with exercise, it is like not giving your pot plants any water, it will wilt and die. Exercise is a crucial part of your daily schedule. The benefits far out weigh the negatives. I know that no extreme training should be done, as you would use up all the required energy to combat and fight the disease. A hear attack would follow. The point I am trying to make is that weight training had been proved beyond doubt to improve general health not break it down.

Wally's way to weight training
Keep the training period short 5-10 min not more. A body builder approach is as follows: You don't train the same body parts every day, give it a 48 hour rest.
Day1   train the chest
Day 2 train shoulders and arms
Day 3 train different body parts
Remember a pot plant gets water twice a week, not daily, it would drown the same with you muscles they will not develop because the are over trained. Basically it's worked out scientifically, from the time of great Reg Parker to Swaznegger and to all practicing body builders of to day. These principles are not kept a secret, but are practiced by millions world wide to improve ill health to good health to better health. In my case is became a savior, a helping hand, a method to get better, a method for the acids and cancer to be driven out. It motivates you to change the body, to change the perspective, a change to change period.

Wally's weight training tips
The quicker the better = High intensity, super setting compounds muscle with specific   muscle lift explosively

10 Tips
1. more salt
2. Eat fish, protein supplements
3. increase water in take
4. stop aerobics
5. lift explosively and quickly
6. rest
7. increase supplements and vitamins
8. eat healthier which gives more power
9. emphasize the negative contraction
10. increase strength thro power lifting, go for low reps.

Use that God given inner power called the Spirit. Don't go negative.
Be prepared to act now don't procrastinate. Move that body now, that spirit is in charge not the body and its negative emotions.

The energy is like a locomotive going at full steam, eyes watchful bright from positive emotions, stand up to your morels and Godly standards, go foreword step by step don't go right or left go straight the narrow way, many people go different ways and take the broad way to hell.

To get better I must have an action plan

1. Make a program for the day.
2. Set out step by step. What is on the schedule?
3. Write down your objectives.
4. They must be attainable
5. What are the objectives?
6. In my case to get better, by removing cancer from my body.
7. Thoughts must be translated into a program action; therefore a daily action plan is necessary.
8. A long distance runner will for example prepare for the comrades, know what you would like to aim for.
9. Preparation is the key word.
10. Make a decision to change.
11. Be honest to yourself.
12. Honor self promises, are the easiest to break but are the most important to be focus on.
13. Focus on the future.
14. Face your fears, the comfort zone, no pain no gain.
15. Take action know. Don't worry about people thoughts, stay focused.
16. Go ahead, don't give up.
17. Break through those barriers they are blessings in disguise, to make me see and be stronger.
18. Take time to recover, renew, motivate rest, take a break, have fun and enjoy quiet time.
19. Be aware of my body and what is going on.
20. What are your mind thoughts?
21. What do you need? Is it time with friends and family, remove too strict deadlines go for those I can attain.
22. Setbacks are opportunities, take advantage of the situation.
23. Make an effort to create enjoyment each day.

Wally's Effort

My thoughts for each day were, that my muscles and blood are connected to the lymph glands, muscle act actively though weight training, the training activates the flowing blood thro the glands fast to the exits and throwing out.

Food for thought

Inactivity **leads to** stagnation **which leads to** cancer spreading silently, deadly.

Wally's thoughts on the cancer attack

Why? Obviously there must be a reason. To purify, by rethinking why I what to live again, the question is it bad or good. If it is good then there is a light at the end of the dark tunnel. But if it is bad there is no hope and a scary death awaits me and by leaving God out of your life this will be your fate. If God is present, there is hope, faith and love burning from HIM to me to all those around me. That does not mean the cancer is gone now but is most definitely going far way faster!

Moments during the day

Plan the day ahead, time, place, to do what. Why? Inactivity is a killer eating away the inside, breaking down not building up, thought need to be carried out. Results, a growing positive result, it is like mighty power sparks becoming flames, flames becoming a great ball of sprouting fire. Let that sprouting fire do its work burning away stress, doubts, pain, lack of faith, sickness, worry for the future, blame on others, the cancer cells eating away at my healthy bones and flesh, will diminish faster. Act by making coffee in the morning for the family. Go down of the floor and do that planned AB crunches, aim for that 200 Max. My next activity is eating roughage to get rid of the night bloating. Drink Pagamisa and calcium pills for extra vitamins needed. Listen to the radio, pulpit, read Nina Smit's messages for the day, read a Psalm. Talk to Martie about the day ahead. What is on the training program for the day, is it training for the legs or arms. Go for it, follow the weight training program now not later the adrenaline pumps the blood flows fast and furious pumping out the enemy cancer.

Thoughts to ponder

What are my new year's resolutions?
They are the big three.
1. Listen to God, the silent voice. Know that silent voice.
2. Listen to others to build up not to break down, therefore now good from evil people.
3. Give myself a change to try again.

Mind control and action give results, rid all wasteful thinking.
Body control and exercise leads to body build up not break down.

Eat right: aim is to eat more bran, protein, veggies, fruit and nuts.
Drink right: aim 2 liters of water daily, it will get rid of waist by controlling water and food intake.

More thoughts

Repent, turn around, regroup, reorganize, redo, and rethink now. Let go, take a different rout to the same destination, of impossible change the destination, change my outlook, change my attitude, and take those donkey blinkers off now. The enemy the cancer is gone now; think it away now, other peoples cancer is not mine, the sun will shine again in my body and soul and spirit. Remember there are others who also care and help don't shut them out, they will get hurt. *Remember charity starts at home.* Therefore my family comes first and is to be defended because it is precious. Life becomes more precious of threatened, so if pain, blood, sweat and tears bear good fruit, Halleluiah to God who made us for a purpose.

A cancer victim: Positive reflections

Break down means to rebuild, to rebuild is more difficult. No one when driving looks all the time in the rear view mirror you look ahead at the road, that's life's story. Chemo has its rebounds but stays a therapy healing, like a burning fire, one day it will burn out, you will live not die, God will decide that not you. Be positive, being negative means walking backwards. Fools are fools because they are arrogant, arrogance brings a fall, the fool is surprised, and will he learn? You will go back to the God who created you. From dust you came to dust you will return your body is expendable, you spirit not it goes on forever.

FIGHT BACK, I am not dead yet.

CANCER has been overcome by many, but my story is my story because your story is different to mine and unique to you only.

The old story known to all is "know yourself" this applies to every cancer victim, a victim because of unknown and unwanted forces determined to take your life. On my side are forces at my disposal which can work for me and you.

The first and foremost is to be positive, you are lost before you start if the initial shock and depression does not wear off.

Positive thoughts: beat cancer

To turn the tide in your favor every successful cancer fighter knows that because your life is at stake, to go onto action fast is the answer, success is near, getting better is near, your life has not ebbed away. Your state of mind is of paramount importance. Your will power, weak, like a weak muscle gets stronger. Empower your will it is you allay in decision making, it is there use it. All great men and women have recognized its building power, to rejuvenate and restore you life to what it was. It is the muscle of the mind. Body builders, swimmers, runners all different sports people use it to make those decisions to get to the top. We as cancer sufferers walk and talk with positive will power to get better. The end result and aim is to be better off after winning to be a changed person, more determined more focused, the old weak self no more, ashes burned out, a bad memory, cancer a forgotten nightmare, because the present counts not the past. If the cancer stays and is overpowering then the great prayer the OUR FATHER is applicable as it says "Our daily bread" Today, now is your focus to find means and ways to overcome. There are people to help you. The doctors, professional helpers at the cancer association your family, the church and close friends, those with other life threatening diseases, those who won and those who give inspiration to go on.

Thoughts during Chemo suffering

What was my greatest enemy?
My greatest enemies are my own insecurities and fears.

What leads us to our downfall?
These insecurities and fears are which leads us in turn to depression, that self made deep black hole.

Pain is that snake biting at us and knowing away at our resistance. So we need a weapon or weapons to fight the enemy. Out greatest source of strength is of Gods spirit in us, our own spirit coming alive and those outside ourselves who assist us. The weapons are, LOVE, FAITH, HOPE for the future, with out pain and suffering, but fun and laughter. I write this because at present it's my fight against cancer, in the past it was broken bones, ruptured in internal organs. With professional help, close family help the insecurity go away, now I know why James: 1 warns us about double mindedness. Two thoughts running parallel and opposites is a sure way to disaster. Single mindedness is the way. It's the way to climb a mountain to win. My thoughts determine my present condition and that in turn determines my future well being. The big word is the NOW and HERE. Thoughts are like many small sparks coming from a fire but disappear into thin air collect those thoughts, bring them into one path and thoughts become action. Action is no enemy, stagnation is one, once the self made fire is burning, thoughts become things becoming what we want positive or negatively to our detriment. Our imagination now takes us to wonderful places of healing, of happiness, where no one can tough us, a dream world.

Therapy means healing. Therapy in the case of drug addicts is action. To force the brain to move away from a habit, activate the body in its own wonderful treasure of power to heal. I have read addicts to get better must, dig holes, break rocks, shock that addicted brain. In the same way move that worn-out body. Don't stop, keep going Paul Said *"run the race, looking forward, don't look back, commit your works to the Lord and your thoughts will be established"* In other words do what you say you are going to do, because it seems as if "self" is the problem child. Alexander the Great said "conquer your self and you conquer the world.

5. Motivation by Example

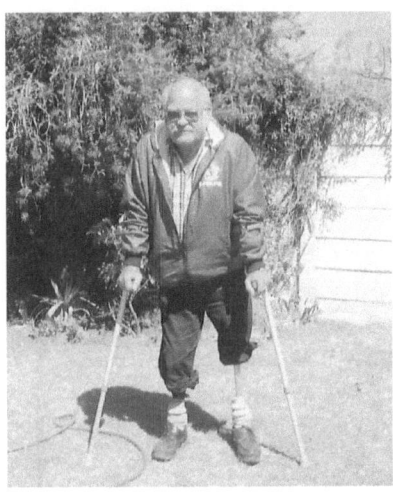

Across the street is a friend of mine by the name of Hendrik. To have sugar diabetes, a heart condition, loose both legs and still be brave is a miracle of faith, hope and courage. Have you got a problem with your motor car? Go to him. You will go to his garage where he is working in the engine, but you won't find him, although he is busy with your car, where is he? You will find him inside the cars bonnet, without his legs on. His strong, steady and sure big hands are busy. The spanner is taking the bots off; his greasy torso turns around and greets you loudly and friendly. His greeting is the traditional "Hoe gaan dit" (How are you). He is under control of the situation; he knows what is wrong with the car. He will give a summary of the problem. When it will go and how much it will cost, very thorough, diplomatic and honest. He will work day and night on the car. He has a good business going, he is well known especially in our street. His other name is "wielietjies" (wheels) because of his way of transport which is a wheel chair. If not in his chair on wheels, he is busily attending to his tuck shop. If he is not at the shop window, calling him, you will hear the clickety-clack of his fast crutches and bionic legs answering you call. He is a man to be admired, a man who leads by example an inspiration to all and to me. He becomes sorrowful when good friends of his with the same problem give up and die. He points to his head and says "Alles is hier bo" (It is all in the mind). The attitude to caner is the same, get better or die. Take action or order your own coffin.

Things to ponder on, from magazine clippings

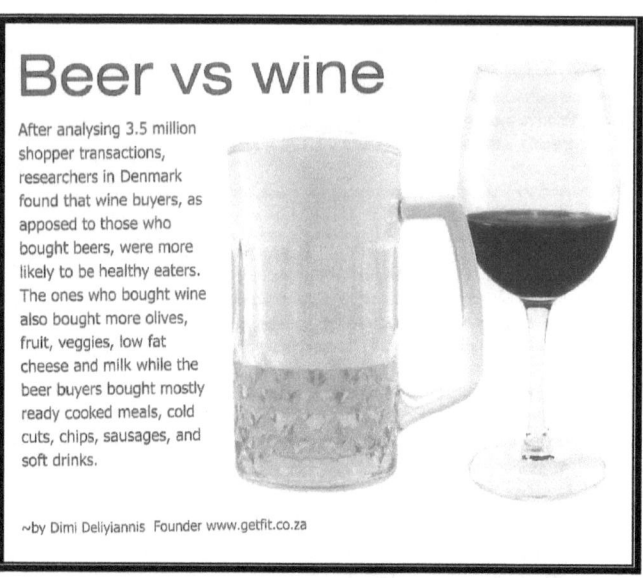

Beer vs wine

After analysing 3.5 million shopper transactions, researchers in Denmark found that wine buyers, as apposed to those who bought beers, were more likely to be healthy eaters. The ones who bought wine also bought more olives, fruit, veggies, low fat cheese and milk while the beer buyers bought mostly ready cooked meals, cold cuts, chips, sausages, and soft drinks.

~by Dimi Deliyiannis Founder www.getfit.co.za

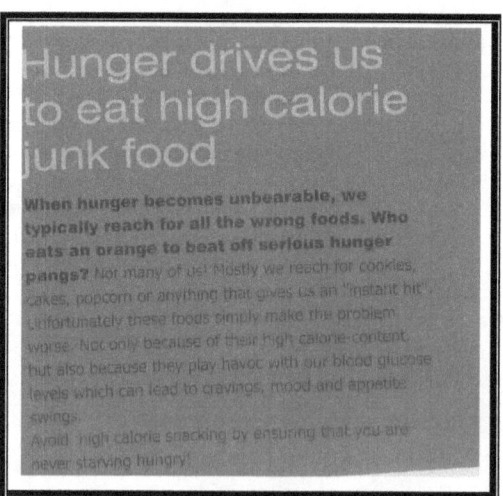

Hunger drives us to eat high calorie junk food

When hunger becomes unbearable, we typically reach for all the wrong foods. Who eats an orange to beat off serious hunger pangs? Not many of us! Mostly we reach for cookies, cakes, popcorn or anything that gives us an "instant hit". Unfortunately these foods simply make the problem worse. Not only because of their high calorie content, but also because they play havoc with our blood glucose levels which can lead to cravings, mood and appetite swings.

Avoid high calorie snacking by ensuring that you are never starving hungry!

Getting it right

SO WHAT DO YOU NEED TO DO TO USE THIS TIME TO BENEFIT YOUR BODY THE MOST?

1) Firstly, drink water. Your body is made up of about 80% water. When you workout, you lose water. This is not only in the form of sweat, but also internally by working tissues. Water is used in the formation of and burning of ATP, and also used to help keep your internal temperature down. Many do not realise the importance of re-hydrating after working out. You can actually lose around 20% of your strength due to dehydration.

You need 4ml of water to store every gram of carbohydrates as glycogen. You also need water to replenish what you lost when you trained. So drink 'till you float. Make sure to spread this water out evenly, as taking in excessive amounts at one time can actually work against you by raising blood pressure and causing your body to release Anti-Diuretic Hormone (ADH), which causes you to excrete more water than you take in.

2) Next is the carbohydrate intake. I explained above why it is so important to consume carbohydrates after working out, but do you know what kind to take in? After training, you want the fastest acting carbohydrate possible. You want it to quickly elevate your blood sugar levels, whilst shuttling nutrients to your muscles. A carbohydrate on the glycemic index scale of 100+ would be optimal. You also want it to be in liquid form for faster absorption. Maltodextrin and dextrose, the carbohydrates used in most creatine sugar mixes and weight gainers are best. Depending on metabolism and the intensity of your workout (we'll assume you train like a madman) you should take in about 1-1.5grams of carbs per kilogram of bodyweight. For a 90kg (200lbs) trainee, that's 100-150 grams of carbs in the post workout period.

3) Many people choose to eat fruit post workout. This is great, but make sure you are eating fruits that are higher in glucose than fructose. Fructose raises blood sugar levels very slowly, and doesn't replenish glycogen stores well. In fact, fructose will only replenish liver glycogen. Try to eat fruits on the higher end of the glycemic index, such as banana's and grapes to ensure a high glucose to fructose ratio.

4) More protein, more protein! Protein is the building block of muscle and there is no denying that. After working out you can absorb and utilise almost 50% more protein than you can at a regular meal. Protein synthesis is highest at this time, so it only makes sense to feed your muscles what they need. A good whey protein would be optimal in this case, since it is broken down into amino acids and absorbed quicker than any other source. I suggest about 30-70grams of protein at this time depending on the size and metabolism of the trainee.

5) Lastly are vitamins and minerals. A good multi vitamin rich in vitamin C and E is optimal at this time. Your cells are oxidised due to free radicals and need these nutrients to help repair muscles and bond due to the damaged caused by these free radicals. Also, chromium and alpha-lipoic acid (ALA) should be taken to make your muscles more insulin sensitive. This allows muscle cells to absorb nutrients much more efficiently.

Now, lets put all this knowledge to good use. Below are a couple of post workout ideas, each are tailored to a hard gainer of 90kg (200 lbs.), so adjust calories to your needs.

6. Nutrition

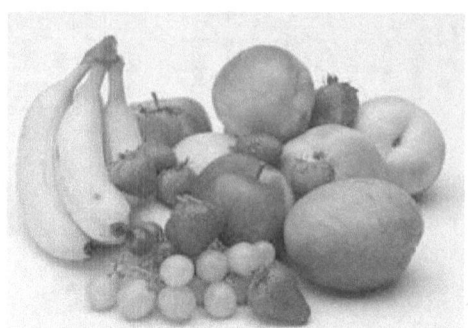

The vitamin E supplement and exercise

Statement: Exercise has only a positive and beneficial effect on the body.
Right...Wrong. According to the author of the book by Dr. K Cooper of the US, "Coopers ant oxidation revolution" it says "The bodies need for O2 during exercise, produces free radicals, which oxidize the fats in the muscle cells called 'n "lipid per oxidation". This process may damage the cells and increase aging. "Over exercise"

Why Vitamin E? Vitamin E has proved to combat cell damage. It assists in the maintenance and upkeep of the lung function. In some cases it serves as a barrier against some types of cancer, thus in effect of keeping the cells healthy. Where is vitamin E found in food?
Example: mealies, wheat germ oil, vegetable oil, almonds, sunflower seeds, walnuts, whole wheat bread and a pill supplement are another option.

It has been well documented that Whey protein powder from scientific research is becoming a common factor in that it is the best protein source nature has to offer. Its immunity connection: It enhances the immunity responses that are compromised by negative elements such as excessive exercise, anabolic, steroids (excessive medication?). Recent studies have shown that whey is superior to egg albumin, casein, soy, beef, and fish. With regard to enhancement of both cellular and hormonal immune responses, such as anti body production or T-cell medicated of B-cells. What may also be of benefit to patients suffering from microbial infections, cancer autoimmune diseases, so it can be concluded that whey and egg are the highest quality source of protein food supplementation, and can be considered to be more than just food for muscle. (Ref: Muscle Evolutions)

Atkins:
Protein: A group of compounds made up of chains of amino acids, needed for growth and repair of human tissues, and provides the body with energy and heat, needed for the manufacture of hormones, antibodies, enzymes, also to maintain acid alkali balances.

Types of Diabetes:

1. Insufficient insulin produced, requiring injections of insulin.
2. More common known as non-insulin dependent more sugar is made than required. A strict diet must be followed cutting out sugar

Weight training

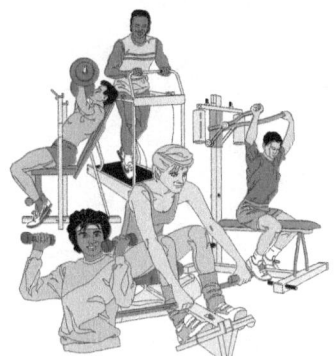

Known as resistance training using weights to develop muscles growth and strength for successful daily healthy living.

Mental health

Post Traumatic Stress Disorder: (Ref: Mental Health center)

Begins after a traumatic event such as hearing about having cancer, it involves a threat, or serious injury or the threat of death diagnosis from a doctor

Reacts by: intense fear and helplessness

THREE GROUPS OF SYMTOMS:

1. Re experiencing traumatic memory (flash backs)
2. Avoidance emotionless, numbness, trying not to think about the bad news (denial)
3. Hyparousal symptoms like irritability, outbursts of anger, noise, food smells, overaggressive behavior

IMPACTS: On the family, the work and anxiety and social disorder

HELP: See your doctor or specialist medication or psychotherapy.

Fiber is a means to get rid of waste in the colon and Leeds to protection against breast and ovular cancer.

7. Dietary Risks

Diet factors that increase the possibility of cancer:

BREAST CANCER: High alcohol intake
High fat intake
Low intake of fruit and vegetables

PANCRAS CANCER: High alcohol intake
High fat intake
Low intake of fruit and vegetables

LUNG CANCER: Low intake of fruit and vegetables

COLON CANCER: Red meat, fat,
Low intake of fruit and vegetables
Alcohol intake

SOMACH CANCER: Low intake of fruit and vegetables
High intake of preserved or smoked food
Low intake of fiber

PROSTRATE CANCER: Fat

MOUTH AND THROAT: Alcohol
Low intake of fruit and vegetables

Ref: A. ELS NUTRITION

8. Atkins

Components of food: protein, fat and carbohydrates

Why protein?
Essential for building and maintaining muscles, bones, organs and tissues, repairing body and muscle damage, some proteins like nuts, seeds, beans, Soya, whole grains, they pair up with other foods to form a complete protein makeup.

Why fat?
Good for you and bad, the good is for storing energy and making hormones. Examples are meat, fish, chicken and veggies.
Bad fat is fatty acids in processed food

Carbohydrates:
Sugars and starches is the quickest source of energy
Good: Unrefined veggies containing minerals, enzymes, and fiber.
Bad: Products not found in nature like sugar, golden syrup, pasta, and white rice, flour.
Bad cabs lead to (unrefined) to epidemics, obesity and diabetes.
Good carbohydrates: fruit and grains.
Bad carbohydrates: the sugar roller coaster if in excess. The good is that it gives energy fast, but too much it is stored as fat or cholesterol in the veins, blood clotting, brain attack or strokes.

Further effects:
Increase in blood sugar, insulin secretion increase blood storage, and low blood sugar low energy too much sugar cravings for more sugar and the vicious circle continues.

Why insulin?
To bring the cells the glucose they need
Keep blood sugar levels normal.

Fiber is your friend

ATKINS MEDICAL SUPPORT

1. Drugs can cause a side effect
2. The right foods through Atkins brings down high blood
3. Lowering effect of blood pressure.
4. Be sure the doctor checks the cholesterol levels to enable you to change your die

MYTHS KETSIS not dangerous

1. Burns fat
2. All butter meat, cheese will raise cholesterol
3. Exercise not necessary – physical activity controls and keeps you slim
4. Too much protein- high protein diet strengthens muscles and bones also by means of calcium intake.
5. Lack of calcium leads to a depletion of protein and calcium resulting in octopuses.

OSTEOPOROSIS

1. Brittle bones with a lack of density
2. Dim perm count
3. Some patients sex diminishes
4. Changes in physical appearance
5. In case of women with breast loss of mastechemy
6. Resulting stress and anxiety
7. Decreased libido
8. Tension
9. Fatigue

The disease causes:

1. Stress
2. Anxiety
3. Drug side effects
4. Inadequate nutrition
5. Sleep
6. Depleted blood counts
7. Fluid intake
8. Pain mane medication
9. Stress medication
10. Mild exercise

MILD EXERCISE

Will decrease fatigue and increase body and muscle activity and in turn increase energy and there for motivation to get better and feel better.

Nutritional support

1. Small regular meals
2. Supplements
3. Stimulants
4. Carbohydrates
5. More protein
6. Avoid smoking
7. Avoid alcohol

Ref: EX: CHEMO THERAPY AND I BY D. LUMLEY

9. Chemo – side effects

HPE

Hand-foot syndrome: Redness, tenderness, burning, tingling, itching in the extremities, blistering.
PREVENTION

1. Tell the doctor or nurse
2. Attention to palms, feet, folds of skin
3. Smear cream or Vaseline
4. Wear loose fitting clothes
5. Avoid vigorous rubbing
6. Unnecessary walking
7. Wear soft shoes
8. Avoid hot water
9. As a precaution take vitamin B6
10. Antiperspirant smearing
11. Hormonal therapy

Certain cancers feed on hormone, which stimulate cancerous growth, breast and the prostrate.

PREVENTION
Hormonal drugs

Side effects:
1. Hot flushes
2. Breast tenderness
3. Tiredness
4. Constipation
5. Weight gain
6. Fluid retention

IMMUNOTHERAPY

Drugs given at home after chemo have been completed.

Side effects:

1. Flu like symptoms
2. Tiredness
3. Loss of appetite
4. Sexually: chemo may cause temporary storability
5. Avoid alcohol
6. Eat softer foods
7. Yogurt
8. Avoid dairy products if allergic to
9. Remove dentures

CONSTIPATION
1. Loss of bowel movement
2. Insufficient fluid intake
3. Incorrect diet
4. Obstruction management: a natural medication
5. Medication
6. Poor bowel habits
7. Lack of intake of either dried fruits, bran fruits

DIARRHEA
1. Tumor
2. Surgery
3. Radiotherapy
4. Stress
5. Facial plug

Management:
1. Medication to stop diaphone
2. Use of Vaseline around rectum
3. Diet adjustment, high proteins, eggs, cheese, fish, chicken, custard, and sago.
4. Fruits – bananas, apples
5. Jungle oats
6. Bread
7. Pasta – macaroni
8. Veggies – carrots, potatoes, spinach, squash

Avoid:
1. Alcohol
2. Smoking
3. Fatty foods
4. Spices

TASTE
Change in taste like
1. Bitterness
2. Meat taste differently
3. New foods new tastes
4. Dislike of certain foods
5. Metallic taste
6. Medical taste

Causes:
1. Excretion of amino – acids gives a bitter taste
2. Tumor in oral cavity, nasal, salivary glands
3. Mouth ulcers
4. Vomiting
5. Smells
6. Poor oral hygiene
7. Poor fitted dentures trap food

BLADDER
Infection of bladder can be caused by chemo and is a side affect

Prevention:

1. Increase fluid intake, water or,
2. Take citron soda to balance chemical balance in urine

Numbness in – or tingling of toes

1. Due again to chemo
2. Cold feeling in front of feet
3. Discolored finger nails

STEATITES (gut)
Inflammatory condition of gastro infest Tina tract

1. It may appear 5 –7 days after chemo
2. Oral hygiene important
3. Visit dentist
4. Avoid spices and acids

10. Why a blood count and hair loss?

Bone marrow play a vital role, they contain cells that have developed into stages of development, reaching maturity and then dying but Chemotherapy inhibit the process of cell division. Blood tests are required at every treatment cycle. Before treatment is done the count must be correct and could cause a delay if not. Until the blood count is right. Most patients feel tired after treatment and will feel listless after a few days. Once the body has secreted the waste cancer cells he will regain energy nutrition. Avoid anxiety, depression, or worries, medication to relax or sleep if the doctor allows it.

SIDE EFFECTS

1. Nausea, vomiting
2. Liver tumor causing a blockage
3. Psychologically
4. Negative information about treatment

COPING

1. Avoid rich foods
2. Use the prescribed medication
3. Eat at intervals
4. Salads, cold foods is easier to manage
5. Dry biscuits
6. Calm yourself

Hair loss

Hair absorbs a certain amount of chemo in the blood stream resulting in hairless. New hair will appear, maybe a bit different in color or texture. Use shampoo. Don't color or perm. Message well, cut hair of if necessary. You can get coverings like wigs, caps or hats.

11. Different Therapies

The different therapy is what every sufferer must go through.

Chemotherapy:

The treatment depends on the origin and grade of the cancer. Various combinations are used depending on the type of cancer. The object of the use of chemical agents is to reach all areas of the body, which contain cancerous cells. The drugs used are decided apron by the oncologist, their side effects and structure. The drugs may interrupt or altar the effects of the cell growth cycle. The cancer cells multiply more rapidly than normal cells, therefore absorbing the chemo and thereby destroying themselves. The combination of drugs is admixture at prescribed interval to allow recovery of toxicity in normal cells.

THREE METHODS OF ADMINISTERING THE DRUGS

1. INTRAMASCULAR: injection to arm of buttocks
2. INTRAVENOUSLY: a needle inserted into the vein
3. BY MOUTH: tablets

Al dosages are individually for your specific needs and body area height and weight. The regularity and duration of the therapy varies with each person, depending on how your body reacts to treatment and the effect on the cancer cells. The medical oncologist monitors constant evaluation of the progress. Surgery or radiotherapy or hormonal therapy might have to be taken in conjunction with the chemo. The physician in charge will explain side effects. The severity depends and varies from person to person, depending on their health and strength. Cut all alcohol and smoking. Carry on with sport; exercise keeps the bodies muscles in shape, as long as it does not exhaust you.

Your Thoughts:

Stay positive, get through the day's treatment.

PHASES

1. Diagnostic
2. Treatment
3. Follow up

Join a group of qualified people to explain and help like sisters, intuitionalist, psychiatrists, priests, doctors, family, and health workers.

DIANOSTIC PHASE:

You are told.
It is traumatic
Absorb the news
Go for treatment
Follow up

FOLLOW UP STAGE: Disease free or remission stage

FINANCIAL FACTORS:

1. Factors – distance to clinic
2. Accommodation
3. Medical aid or government
4. Work loss and pay loss
5. Child care at home
6. Food
7. Clothing
8. Gifts

12. Wat is Kanker?

2.1 ALGEMENE INLIGTING

Kanker is 'n baie ou bekende siekte. Daar bestaan bewyse dat die primitiewe mens ook as gevolg van kanker gely het. Jare gelede was dit 'n siekte wat groot vrees veroorsaak het omdat kanker 'n gewisse dood beteken het.

Vandag hoor ons meer van kanker omdat ons meer omtrent die siekte weet. Dokters kan nou kanker vroeër opspoor en diagnoseer. Tydige behandeling kan die lewens van baie individue red wat andersins nie sou oorleef het nie.

Omdat die lewensverwagting deesdae langer is en kanker meer dikwels by ouer mense voorkom, lyk dit asof kanker toeneem en meer algemeen voorkom. Dit is beslis so dat baie oorsake van kanker aan die moderne leefwyse toegeskryf kan word. Sommige oorsake is van nature in die omgewing, maar word gevaarlik wanneer dit misbruik word; ander is kunsmatig en is die skeppings en newe-produkte van 'n moderne nywerheidsgemeenskap.

Kanker kom nie algemeen voor by jongmense nie. Dit is nietemin belangrik vir 'n jongmens om van kleins af van die siekte te leer om sodoende homself en sy familie te bevoordeel.

2.1 NORMALE SELLE

'n Huis word gebou van klein deeltjies wat stene, blokke hout, klippe of ander boumateriaal kan wees.

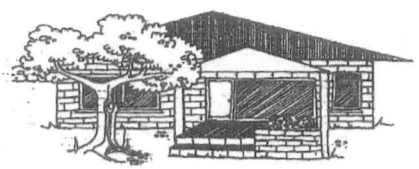

Op dieselfde manier is menslike wesens, diere en plante ook uit baie klein deeltjies wat selle genoem word, opgebou. Hierdie selle is so klein dat dit slegs deur 'n mikroskoop gesien kan word. Ons moet besef dat die menslike liggaam uit baie verskillende tipe selle opgebou is (miljoene van hulle) - ten minste 300

vir die uitvoering van sy taak en elkeen verrig een of meer funksies om die hele liggaam te help. Spierselle is byvoorbeeld lank en dun en verkort om 'n gewrig te buig; selle wat vet berg, bevat 'n sakkie olie; en velselle beskerm die buitekant van die liggaam.

Alhoewel hierdie selle van mekaar verskil in vorm en funksie, benodig hulle dieselfde basiese bestanddele om hul funksies te kan uitvoer. Selle leef nie vir ewig nie. Hulle sterf en word deur ander vervang. Die proses waardeur nuwe selle gemaak word, is *selverdeling*. Normale selverdeling is 'n orderlike proses. In teenstelling is kankerselverdeling 'n abnormale, wanorderlike en onbeheerde proses.

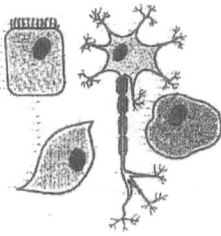

'n Sel is baie slim. Dit wil amper voorkom asof 'n sel kan dink. Dit is egter nie moontlik nie omdat die sel te klein is om 'n brein te kan hê. Die sel bevat egter 'n "rekenaar" wat al sy aktiwiteite beheer. Wat belangrik is, is dat alle selle in die liggaam drie baie belangrike reëls gehoorsaam:

REËL NO. 1 - DOEN WAT JY VERONDERSTEL IS OM TE DOEN. Dit beteken dat elke sel 'n spesifieke funksie het. 'n Breinsel kan nie been maak nie en 'n beensel kan nie dink nie. Elke sel het sy eie werk.

ReëL NO. 2 - BLY OP JOU PLEK. Dit beteken dat verskillende selle nie sommer na willekeur kan rondbeweeg in die liggaam nie. Lewerselle bly in die lewer en breinselle bly in die brein. Die enigste selle wat toegelaat word om rond te beweeg is die rooibloed- en witbloedselle. Ook die vroulike eiersel kan na bevrugting 21 cm weg beweeg van die eierstok (ovarium) af na die baarmoeder (uterus) toe. Behalwe vir hierdie selle moet alle ander selle op hul plekke bly.

Reël NO. 3 - VERDEEL NET WANNEER NODIG. Dit is 'n baie belangrike reël. Alle selle kan verdeel, maar hulle moet "weet" wanneer om te verdeel en ook, baie belangrik, wanneer om nie te verdeel nie. As selle sommer so ongekontroleerd verdeel, sou die liggaam net 'n opeengehoogte klomp selle gewees het en dit kan nie so wees nie.

Hoe maak 'n sel seker dat hierdie 3 GOUE REËLS gehoorsaam en uitgevoer word? Hoe word die sel beheer? Deur 'n klein rekenaartjie wat DNS genoem word en in die kern/nukleus van elke sel aangetref word.

2.3   KANKERSELLE

Soms gaan iets met die kern van die sel verkeerd en ontvang die sel 'n verkeerde boodskap. Dit staan bekend as *mutasie*. Die sel word dan nie die spesifieke sel wat dit veronderstel is om te wees nie, maar in plaas daarvan bly dit eenvoudig en kan nie die korrekte funksie uitvoer nie. Dit is gebeur selde, maar wanneer dit wel gebeur, ontstaan 'n kankersel. Hierdie sel verdeel aanhoudend, maar is **buite normale beheer** en vorm 'n klein groepie eenvoudige selle in plaas van spesiale selle. Die kankersel begin 'n *gewas/groeisel* vorm. Soos wat die groepe selle groei, versprei dit tussen die omringende normale selle en beskadig hulle. Hierdie verspreiding van kankerselle word *infiltrasie* genoem.

Gewasse kan dodelik of onskadelik wees. Onskadelike gewasse kan inmeng met liggaamlike funksies en moet chirurgies verwyder word, maar dit versprei nie na ander dele van die liggaam nie. In die meeste gevalle is hierdie tipe gewasse nie lewensgevaarlik nie omdat dit nie na ander dele van die liggaam versprei nie.

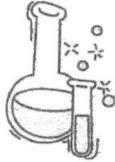

Dodelike gewasse dring gesonde weefsel binne en vernietig dit. Selle van hierdie gewasse kan van die oorspronklike gewas afbreek en dan deur middel van die bloed- of limfsisteem na ander dele van die liggaam versprei. Hierdie manier van verspreiding word *metastase* genoem.

Kanker is dus 'n groep siektes waar daar ongekontroleerde groei van abnormale selle plaasvind en wat die vermoë het om te kan versprei. Dit beteken om meer kankeragtige gewasse elders in die liggaam te vorm. Die selle in hierdie sekondêre gewasse (metastases) is dieselfde as die in die primêre gewas. Borskanker wat na die lewer versprei, word dus "metastatiese borskanker" genoem, en die pasiënt word vir borskanker en nie vir lewerkanker nie behandel.

Die verspreiding van kanker kan tot een orgaan beperk word, of dit kan ver weg beweeg van die oorspronklike gewas af. Laasgenoemde tipe kanker word gewoonlik met laer oorlewingsyfers geassosieer. Dit is waarom vroeë opsporing en behoorlike behandeling - voordat die kanker versprei - so belangrik is.

OPSOMMING

- Die menslike liggaam is opgebou uit ten minste 300 verskillende tipe selle.

- 'n Sel is so klein dat dit nie met die blote oog gesien kan word nie.

- Die liggaam bestaan uit biljoene selle.

- Elke sel gehoorsaam 3 fundementele reëls: "Doen wat jy moet doen", "Verdeel net indien nodig", en "Bly op jou plek".

- Kanker begin met 'n klein selletjie.

- 'n Sel word beheer deur 'n "rekenaar" wat DNS genoem word.

- Mutasies word deur chemikalieë en bestraling veroorsaak.

- Kritieke mutasies kan veroorsaak dat die sel onophoudelik verdeel. So vorm dit 'n gewas.

- Kankerselle verbreek dus die reël wat sê "Verdeel net indien nodig".

- Kankerselle gaan verder: hulle verbreek ook die reël wat sê "Bly op jou plek". Hulle bly nie op hulle plek nie. Hulle versprei deur die liggaam. Dit word metastase genoem en is dodelik.

- Die beste manier om die individu se lewe te red is om die kanker te verwyder voordat metastase plaasvind.

2.4 WAT VEROORSAAK KANKER?

Daar bestaan nog nie presies sekerheid oor wat die oorsaak is dat selle buite beheer raak en kankerselle vorm nie. Navorsing is tans besig om op verskeie moontlike areas te fokus.

Sommige tipes kanker kom algemeen voor in sommige families; daarom is navorsers besig om na leidrade in die gene van lede van hierdie families te soek. Gene bevat die oorerflikheidskode wat van een sel na die volgende sel oorgedra word, en dus ook van ouer na kind. Sover bekend, kan slegs een tipe kanker - 'n baie rare oogkanker (retinoblastoom)- as oorerflik beskou word. 'n Familiegeskiedenis van sekere tipes kanker word egter as 'n risikofaktor beskou.

2.4.1 OMGEWINGSFAKTORE

Ongeveer 80% van alle kanker hou verband met gedragsfaktore of omgewingsfaktore - ons dieet, of ons rook of oormatig drink of nie, die lug wat ons inasem, blootstelling aan chemikalieë of oormatige blootstelling aan die son. Geeneen van ons beskik oor die vermoë om oorerflikheidsfaktore wat ons selstruktuur beïnvloed te beheer nie, maar ons het almal 'n groot mate van beheer oor gedrags- of omgewingsfaktore.

2.4.2 KARSINOGENE

'n Karsinogeen is 'n stof wat kanker in mense kan inisieer of bevorder (dus kankerwekkende stowwe). Hierdie stowwe is geïdentifiseer deur middel van studies met diere en ook bevolkingstudies van mense as stowwe wat 'n statisties betekenisvolle toename in kanker-insidensie kan veroorsaak.

CHEMIESE AGENTE - Chemikalieë wat kanker veroorsaak, sluit koolwaterstowwe, seker metale, medikasies en hormone in. Koolwaterstowwe is bestanddele van sigaretrook wat longkanker veroorsaak. Arseen word gebruik in insekdoders, die vervaardiging van glas en keramiek en ook in die smelting van erts. Ander chemikalieë wat in industriële prosesse gebruik word, soos bv. nafta-samestellings, kan tot blaas- en lewerkanker aanleiding gee. Hoë vlakke oestrogeen word ook geassosieer met die voorkoms van kanker van die baarmoeder (uterus).

BIOLOGIESE AGENTE - Organismes wat kanker veroorsaak, sluit virusse, bakterieë en ook multisellige parasiete in. Die belangrikste menslike kanker wat met 'n virusinfeksie verband hou is lewerkanker wat na hepatitis B

virusinfeksie volg. Virusse word ook met leukemia geassosieer. 'n Tipe blaaskanker wat veral in Egipte voorkom, word deur klein bloedparasiete veroorsaak.

Die Menslike Immuniteitsgebrek Virus (MIV) word met die Verworwe Immuniteitsgebrek Sindroom (VIGS) geassosieer. Pasiënte met MIV lei aan 'n verbrokkeling van hulle natuurlike immuniteitsisteem. Een van die siektes waaraan VIGS pasiënte kan lei, is Kaposi se Sarkoom, 'n tipe kanker wat in die sagte weefsel van die velmembrane wat die liggaam se organe omring, voorkom. Om VIGS te hê kan 'n risikofaktor vir kanker wees, maar VIGS is nie kanker nie.

FISIESE AGENTE - Ultraviolet en hoë-energie radiasie is ook karsinogene. Oormatige blootstelling aan die son se ultravioletstrale is die primêre oorsaak van velkanker. Die gebruik van sonlampe of sonbeddens, wat ook van ultravioletstrale gebruik maak, kan ook tot oormatige blootstelling lei. Diagnostiese x-strale word versigtig gebruik sodat die persoon nie oormatig blootgestel word nie. Asbestos is 'n kristal wat ingeasem word en die voering van die longe irriteer wat dan tot longkanker aanleiding kan gee.

2.5 HOE PERSOONLIKE GEDRAGSPATRONE DIE RISIKO VAN KANKER KAN BEÏNVLOED

'n Kanker risikofaktor is iets wat die moontlikheid het om kanker te kry verhoog. 'n Persoon se risiko om kanker te kry hou direk verband met sy of haar vermoë om karsinogene te vermy, 'n behoorlike dieet te volg, en om opvoeding ontvang rakende die voorkoming van kanker, uit te leef. Ons kan die risiko om kanker te kry verminder deur die risikofaktore te vermy - nie rook nie, geen oormatige blootstelling aan die son - en om positiewe stappe te doen wat die liggaam kan help om homself teen kanker te beskerm. Hierdie stappe sluit 'n goed-gebalanseerde dieet in wat uit min vet en genoeg vesel, vars groente en vrugte bestaan.

2.6 DIE BEHANDELING VAN KANKER

Daar is drie algemene tipes behandeling teen kanker - chirurgie, chemoterapie en radioterapie (bestraling). Sommige behandelingsprogramme kombineer twee of meer van hierdie metodes.

Chirurgie - Die diagnose van kanker word bevestig met 'n mikroskopiese ondersoek van 'n monster van die verdagte selle deur 'n patoloog. Die chirurgiese verwydering van 'n deeltjie van die verdagte gewas word 'n biopsie genoem. Indien die biopsie toon dat die gewas dodelik is, word behandeling onmiddellik begin. Selfs as die gewas

- 133 -

onskadelik is, word dit gewoonlik chirurgies verwyder na afloop van die biopsie.

Chirurgiese verwydering van kanker is die oudste vorm van behandeling. Gewoonlik word die gewas en die omringende weefsel uitgesny. In sommige gevalle waar die kanker deur die hele weefsel of orgaan versprei het, word die hele orgaan verwyder.

Indien die kanker reeds na ander organe versprei en nuwe gewasse (metastases) gevorm het, word die primêre kanker chirurgies verwyder terwyl die sekondêre gewasse met ander vorms van terapie behandel word.

Gedurende die afgelope paar jaar bestaan daar 'n neiging om meer konserwatiewe chirurgie toe te pas - dit beteken dat daar gepoog word om so veel as moontlik van die omringende weefsel en die orgaan waarin die kanker voorkom te red. Op hierdie wyse is nuwe tegnieke ontwikkel om baie vroue met borskanker die grootste deel van hul bors te laat behou. Wanneer kanker met behulp van hierdie minder radikale chirurgiese metodes behandel word, word dit gewoonlik gekombineer met ander vorms van terapie.

Chemoterapie - Chemoterapie is die behandeling van kankerselle met middels wat kanker beveg. Dit word dikwels in kombinasie met chirurgie of in die plek van chirurgie gebruik, of in die geval van algemene kankers wat nie verwyder kan word sonder om die omliggende organe of liggaamsisteme te beskadig nie. Chemoterapie is ook effektief om kankers te beveg wat deur die hele liggaam teenwoordig is, veral leukemie en limfoom.

Radioterapie (bestraling) - Radioterapie behels die behandeling van kankerselle met gammastrale deur middel van kobalt 60 of x-strale. Radioterapie kan ook gebruik word om die grootte van die kankergewas te verminder voordat dit verwyder word, of om die oorblywende kankerselle na chirurgie te vernietig. Dit is ook nuttig om gewasse wat weer voorkom, te laat krimp. 'n Groot probleem wat met radioterapie verband hou, is die toediening van bestraling in veilige dosisse - genoeg om die kankerselle te vernietig, maar nie so baie dat dit die gesonde weefsel beskadig nie.

2.7   NEWE-EFFEKTE VAN KANKERBEHANDELING

Die reaksie op kankerbehandeling verskil baie, maar newe-effekte kan moegheid, gebrek aan eetlus, naarheid, diaree, gedeeltelike of algehele haarverlies en ook emosionele probleme insluit.

Maniere waarop newe-effekte verlig en/of verminder kan word, sluit in:

- Genoegsame rus.

- 'n Gesonde eetplan.

- Fisieke aktiwiteit (gereelde oefening), indien moontlik.

- Ondersteuningsgroepe wat mense help om hul gevoelens te deel en probleme op te los.

2.8   DIE WAARDE VAN VROEë OPSPORING

Die vroeë opsporing van kanker sluit in onmiddellike optrede na simptome en waarskuwingstekens verskyn, roetine-ondersoeke en kanker-ondersoeke (check-ups). Vroeë opsporing verbeter nie net die kanse op oorlewing nie, maar beteken ook minder drastiese en duur behandelingskedules en verminder ook die langtermyn newe-effekte.

2.8.1.   LET OP DIE WAARSKUWINGSTEKENS

Leer jou liggaam ken sodat jy veranderinge onmiddellik sal raaksien. Kanker se waarskuwingstekens is maklik om te onthou. Elkeen van hulle kan verband hou met spesifieke kankers:

- Verandering in 'n vratjie of moesie (vel)

- 'n Seer wat nie wil genees nie (vel, lip, mond, tong en vulva)

- Ongewone bloeding of afskeiding (bors, serviks, ovarium, prostaat, long, blaas, kolon, maag, uterus, leukemie, lewer, pankreas, nier)

- Verdikking of knop (nier, bors, testikel, skildklier, mond, keel, larinks, vulva)

- Slegte spysvertering of probleme om te kan sluk (oesofagus, larinks, skildklier)

- Aanhoudende hoes of heserigheid (long, oesofagus, larinks)

- Wesenlike verandering in maag- of blaasgewoontes (blaas, maag, kolon, prostaat, ovarium)

Onverklaarbare gewigsverlies kan ook 'n aanduiding wees van kankers soos limfoom, leukemie, oesofagus, nier, maag, long of kolonkanker.

Alhoewel hierdie tekens nie altyd kanker beteken nie, is dit altyd wenslik om jou dokter te spreek indien hierdie tekens langer as twee weke aanhou.

Hou jou kinders dop aangesien kanker spesiale waarskuwingstekens vir hulle het:

- Aanhoudende koors

- Gereelde pyn wat nie verdwyn nie

- Oggendnaarheid

- 'n Abnormale knop, bv. in die maag of nek

- Blou kolle (bloeding onder die vel)

- Bleek voorkoms (gepaard met lusteloosheid, koors en onverklaarbare blou kolle)

- Veranderinge in balans, beweging of persoonlikheid

- Verandering in die oë, bv. skeelheid

- Versteurde gelaatstrekke

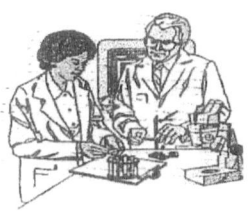

2.8.2 SELFONDERSOEKE KAN DIE VERSKIL VAN 'N LEEFTYD BETEKEN

'n Hele paar kankers kan op 'n afstand gehou word deur middel van gereelde selfondersoeke. Leer jou liggaam ken en wees opmerksaam. Raadpleeg jou dokter sodra jy die eerste tekens raaksien - dit stel jou dokter in staat om op te tree wanneer die kanker hoogs behandelbaar is. Selfondersoeke sluit in ondersoeke van die bors, testikels en vel.

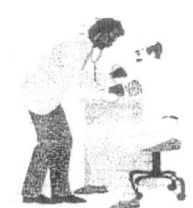

2.8.3 GEREELDE MEDIESE ONDERSOEKE MAAK VAN JOU 'N WENNER

Die mediese wetenskap het alreeds ondersoeke beskikbaar gestel wat baie kankers vroeg kan opspoor, wat dan ook effektiewe behandeling verseker. Dit is veral van toepassing op kanker van die serviks, bors, kolon en prostaat.

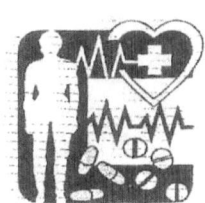

Chapter 6

Reflections, Prayers and Motivation

Chapter 6   Reflections, Prayers and Motivations

Title   **Page**

Reflections

Reflect on the past and the future

Reform yourself

Refrain from further bodily abuse

Refresh yourself

Take refuge in Jawe God

Use your families love to build up

Re enforce your will power

Be strong

Reject evil

Rejoice in the good

Rejuvenate your self

Don't re lapse

Forgive and forget

Relate to good

Master your bad habits

Repent

Turn around

Reroute your forces

Don't abuse yourself

Rebuild yourself

Forgive injury you will be healed

Don't looks back look foreword?

Reward the good I do

Revise my plans

Control my thoughts

Organize myself

Plan ahead

Lead yourself to health control your health, it is my life

Thought control it will bring success and health

Resurrect yourself from the valley of the dead

Be rich in the spirit

Avoid the love of money it's a false god

Be righteous not self righteous

Aim for the straight and the narrow to life

Keep the commandments they lead to life

No pain no gain Christ suffered for gain

Rebuild my broken body and spirit

Change for the good

Rebuke the past, look to the future

Forget the past

Recall the good

Reclaim your rights for yourself

Recreate your mind it is a power

Use your will power it is there for a purpose

Re educate yourself don't stagnate

Start again now the operating word

Revise your strategy often

Resolve to try again and again

Resort to the use of wisdom it's an ally

Repel eve evil and Satan

Save whets left and go on

Retain your sanity

Stone by stone move that mountain, not faith alone.

Family is precious reunite differences a

Restore my moral

Rebuild

Refrain from insincerity get sincerity

Be saint aim for perfection

Restore your dignity become healthy again

Retreat from what you can't do, do what you can do

Return to God your maker

Honor your parents they did support you.

Reunite yourself to your self, do not eject yourself

Revenge is loss, start again

Reverse the past nothing is impossible

Revise the future, think big

Plan ahead strategies each day is precious

Revue your enemy Satan now, he is the father of lye's

Revolt against your weak body, strengthen it now

Love your brother, otherwise hell waits

It may bring you down it is weak

Don't let wild emotions run my life they are false- and burn out quickly

They are like a river that runs dry

Revive your flagging spirits

Revolutionize my thoughts they are mighty, starting from a small spark, to a fireball

Directing your life

Use your sub conscious, it's your friend in need.

Be in charge don't let sin rule you.

Prayers

The fire on the altar must never go out. Leviticus 6:13

The fire on the altar is our faith, which never goes out. The priest had the responsibility then, but now it is ours to maintain that burning in our hearts.

The bible refers to fellowship offerings, in our case means love for our fellow man, a prerequisite for faith and love according to Paul in Corinthians 13.

Stop giving that faithful in put self and sacrifice and your faith will be like that fire gone out, cold and unfeeling to yourself and to others and ultimately to God himself. How can I go back to him if I have rejected him?   God says do not give up, and pray always, meaning carry on regardless, don't worry about that recurring sin and weakness because God's son died on the cross for it. So by keeping the faith by having your eyes in him, there won't be a problem rekindling it daily.

His son said, "that by looking at the cross, lifted up you will be saved!" He will honour you for that small sacrifice just by looking.

Know that can't be so difficult.

Eternal life

"Eternal life means knowing God and knowing Jesus whom he sent" John 17:3

Seek constant contact with him; he is the life's flow through the spirit, mind, and body. He restores, renews, cleans and heals by doing it in action and by achieving its object.

Noiseless He draws near.

Be still, I am here.

The son of God needs time to communicate with his father, God to all.

When you are weak that you are strong because he takes over, power comes from shutting yourself away with him, his quiet time. Rely on him alone, he is the supplier.

Face your responsibilities.

Pray that what goes wrong goes right again, banish that evil, you have that power to do so!

God is your helper from weakness to power, sin to salvation, insecurity to security, poverty to plenty, cold in different to love, and giving from unforgiving resentment to perfect forgiveness.

Don't be satisfied with other peoples faith, where is your own faith?

He will guide my efforts, he is not punishing you for your sins, he did for them, and I am the one to repent and turn around and am replenished.

Eternal life is a gift from Him!

Regret nothing

Regret noting, not even all your sins and failures.
When you see the earths great wonders from that mountain height, you don't spend you time worrying about how you fell and fainted on the stumbling stones on the way up, breath in that refreshing cold air.

Breathing the rich blessings of each new day, forget all that lies behind, man is made to carry the weight of one day- 24 hours- no more, if he is weighed down with the weight of years past, and the day ahead his back breaks.

I, Jesus, have promised to help you with the burden of one day only, the past I have taken from you, but if you foolish hearts carry that extra burden, then you mock me and my cross and you mock me of you think I must share it. Whether it was a good or bad day and it is ended, what remains it be lived is that next 24 hours, face it when you awake.

A man on a long walk carries only what he needs, would you pity him if you saw him bearing the overwhelming weight of past walks or marches, worn out shoes, worn out uniforms, bent backs, yet in the mental and spiritual life you and me do the same.

Let's rejuvenate our selves again by shaking off the past by looking at him and praising his name Jawe, again and again.

Amen

What YAWE Says?

Pray until you almost stop, because trust has become so rock like you, pray on because it has become such a habit you can't resist it.
Pray merges into Praise.
Your attitude is show by your love and laughter.
Look within, there is your power.
Look and be saved, keep looking, a power and peace flows beyond all understanding.
Surely it is in the power of any one to look.
Look and keep looking and doubt flee.
Lay hold of the truth; affirm it, like holding firmly on to a rope pulling you to safety.
How foolish are your attempts to save yourself, if you hold on with one hand and hold on with the other, try swimming on your own.
You are hindering the person helping you.
Obey my commands.
They are steps that lead to success.
Keep calm, unmoved.
Go back to that silent time with me to recover; you will accomplish more to recover this calmness than on all your own efforts.
My task are not inadequate so don't feel in adequate, so don't block that channel, my spirit must work in.
Yourself is in the way,
Pray about it.
Accomplish one thing at a time; until your goal is met then go on.
I am watching over you.
All is well.
Strength is provided hourly and daily.
The fault, the sin is yours; ask forgiveness otherwise you will fail for the lack of that effort by you.
Tender love is the secret.
Train yourself to love your neighbour, and not to hate yourself as Yawe himself made you in his likeness.

A few don'ts
Don't have hate or resentment.
Have patients.
God is love; you have his power and supply of all your needs.
There do my will.
Then there will be no barriers between me and you.
Remember unbelief is a barrier.

Is love a crime?
Let me do the fighting for you, the combating evil for you, persevere in my will, accept my discipline, and as the scripture says"your joy no man can take from you"
Daily happenings don't just happen. What may seem to be a coincidence is really my love for thought.

YAWE God's will

For you and me - The key

Acceptance, this will bring happiness and holiness and divine revelation. This yoke of acceptance is the way of the cross, because at its foot the heaviness of sin, suffering, desires, failures, pain sufferings are taken.

What is Gods will?
Each task, work, how big or small become a divine interest accept it, give thanks for it.

Repeat it daily, it will become a strengthening habit.

Results?
Transformation of that rebellious self, a change, your cry is always heard.
God hears it, but man does not hear his response, man not hearing or failing to hear, or make an effort to listen, remains unsaved, helped.
You are not the only one who was lonely, Jesus was deserted by his friends, but in forgiveness he gave them the power to become his children, the power to heal, forgive and heal.

Why, because only when you have realized your error, you have learned to become humble, the key to Yawe God will.

What are our greatest stumbling blocks?
Trust

Be like Abraham who was willing to kill his own son as a sacrifice for the unseen.
This is the final test, relaying on God alone, his will alone, that unseen spirits force which, "you can't eat bread alone, without Gods breath" that is his will and life for you and me.

The secret of spiritual prosperity

Know God

Look to no other

See no other supply

Then you will be saved

Regard me as your only supply

What you need, ask me?

What others need, look to me?

Claim, claim, claim.

Remember I fed the Israelites through the desert, wilderness, lack of food and lack of water, those who lacked discipline fell, those who had trusting faith made it to Canaan, the land of milk and honey.

You and me, must decide now, trust in the Lord and be led or be like some of them, losers(an extract from the book "God calling")

The two listeners, the theme coming from the prophet Isaiah "look t me all of you to be saved"

We are who we are!

Our thoughts control us.

This is the main reason for success or failure, why, because strong positive thoughts make strong positive people, weak negative thoughts make weak negative people, people, week negative thoughts make weak negative people, because these aristocrat's weak forces, just as strong and concentrated forces are in the mind are just as strong and concentrated and weak flames are like list sparks, lost forever.

This same law of nature works for us in our thoughts. Do I allow these forces to work for me or against it!

It is the major part of me, the unseen, almighty muscle, the beat of my heart, my life's blood, these thoughts!

Do I let these thoughts take change of me, so that I become like that complaining howling unsatisfied dog in the night?

A direct result of my thought are my lack, lack of money, work, faith, hope, health, but the big surprise is that there is hope through reassuringly no matter what the circumstances past or present.

If you feed your thoughts like a master gardener his garden with devotion love, and attention, the results will be a rich harvest of success, or neglect will result

In life's failures, means if you don't making an effort it will go very badly for you because the little you have will be taken away, but what you are going to do today and in so thinking what you have decided, will happen.

Our lessons take control of your greatest gift, your thoughts, by means of will power, self knowledge, and lasting the prophets call wisdom!

Bibliography
Proverbs   16.3
Luke   19 - 26
Mind control by John Kehoe.

MY SON

This is great, take a moment to read it, it will make your day!
The ending will surprise you.

Take my Son

A wealthy man and his son loved to collect rare works of art. They
everything in their collection, from Picasso to Raphael. They would
together and admire the great works of art.
When the Vietnam conflict broke out, the son went to war. He was
courageous and died in battle while rescuing another soldier. The fa
notified and grieved deeply for his only son.
About a month later, just before Christmas, there was a knock at th
young man stood at the door with a large package in his hands.
He said, "Sir, you don't know me, but I am the soldier for whom you
gave his life. He saved many lives that day, and he was carrying me
when a bullet struck him in the heart and he died instantly. He ofte
about you, and your love for art." The young man held out this pack
know this isn't much. I'm not really a great artist, but I think your
would have wanted you to have this."
The father opened the package. It was a portrait of his son, painted
young man. He stared in awe at the way the soldier had captured th
personality of his son in the painting. The father was so drawn to t
that his own eyes welled up with tears. He thanked the young man
offered to pay him for the picture. "Oh, no sir, I could never repay u
son did for me. It's a gift."
The father hung the portrait over his mantle. Every time visitors ca
home he took them to see the portrait of his son before he showed th
the other great works he had collected.
The man died a few months later. There was to be a great auction o
paintings. Many influential people gathered, excited over seeing the
paintings and having an opportunity to purchase one for their colle
On the platform sat the painting of the son. The auctioneer
pounded his gavel. "We will start the bidding with this pict

the son. Who will bid for this picture?"

There was silence.

Then a voice in the back of the room shouted, "We want to see the f paintings. Skip this one."

But the auctioneer persisted. "Will somebody bid for this painting. ' start the bidding? $100, $200?"

Another voice angrily. "We didn't come to see this painting. We can the Van Goghs, the Rembrandts. Get on with the real bids!"

But still the auctioneer continued. "The son! The son! Who'll take t Finally, a voice came from the very back of the room. It was the lon gardener of the man and his son. "I'll give $10 for the painting." Bei man, it was all he could afford.

"We have $10, who will bid $20?"

"Give it to him for $10. Let's see the masters."

"$10 is the bid, won't someone bid $20?"

The crowd was becoming angry. They didn't want the picture of the They wanted the more worthy investments for their collections.

The auctioneer pounded the gavel. "Going once, twice, SOLD for $1 A man sitting on the second row shouted, "Now let's get on with th collection!"

The auctioneer laid down his gavel. "I'm sorry, the auction is over."

"What about the paintings?"

"I am sorry. When I was called to conduct this auction, I was told stipulation in the will. I was not allowed to reveal that stipulation this time. Only the painting of the son would be auctioned. Whoeve that painting would inherit the entire estate, including the paintin The man who took the son gets everything!"

God gave His son 2,000 years ago to die on the cross. Much like the auctioneer, His message today is: "The son, the son, who'll take the Because, you see, whoever takes the Son gets everything.

Please send this to ten people and back to the one who sent it to yo Do whatever you like, but remember that maybe "one" of the people might have taken the time to send this to, may be just the person wi to hear this message.

You have a choice to make."

PHANTOM PAIN

Amputees often experience some sensation of a phantom limb. Somewhere, locked in their brains, a memory lingers of the nonexistent hand or leg. Invisible toes curl, imaginary hands grasp things, a "leg" feels so sturdy a patient may try to stand on it.

For a few, the experience includes pain. Doctors watch helplessly, for the part of the body screaming for attention does not exist.

One such patient was my medical school administrator, Mr. Barwick, who had a serious and painful circulation problem in his leg but refused to allow the recommended amputation.

As the pain grew worse, Barwick grew bitter.

"I hate it! I hate it!" he would mutter about the leg. At last he relented and told the doctor, "I can't stand it anymore. I'm through with that leg. Take it off." Surgery was scheduled immediately.

Before the operation, however, Barwick asked the doctor, "What do you do with legs after they're removed?"

"We may take a biopsy or explore them a little bit, but afterwards we incinerate them," the doctor replied.

Barwick proceeded with a bizarre request: "I would like you to preserve my leg in a pickle jar. I will install it on my mantle shelf. Then, as I sit in my armchair, I will taunt that leg, 'Hah! You can't hurt me anymore!'"

Ultimately, he got his wish. But the despised leg had the last laugh. Barwick suffered phantom limb pain of the worst degree. The wound healed, but he could feel the torturous pressure of the swelling as the muscles cramped, and he had no prospect of relief. He had hated the leg with such intensity that the pain had unaccountably lodged permanently in his brain.

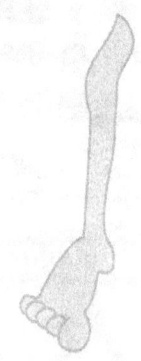

To me, phantom limb pain provides wonderful insight into the phenomenon of false guilt. Christians can be obsessed by the memory of some sin committed years ago. It never leaves them, crippling their ministry, their devotional life, their relationship with others. They live in fear that someone will discover their past. They work overtime trying to prove to God they're truly repentant. They erect barriers against the enveloping, loving grace of God.

Unless they experience the truth in 1 John 3:19-20 that "God is greater than our conscience," they become as painful as poor Mr. Barwick, shaking his fist in fury at the pickled leg on the mantle.

ARNOLD PRATER'S BEST PRIZE ROSE

Arnold Prater, in his book YOU CAN HAVE JOY! tells about a man in a little English village named John Deckard. He was a clerk in a textile factory. A modest and quiet man, he lived in an ordinary little house at the edge of town with his wife and his six-year-old son, Rob. Like thousands of Englishmen, every morning John put on his plain tweed suit, got on his bicycle, and rode to work. Returning home at five in the evening, he would work in his garden until suppertime. Then he would spend a quiet evening with his pipe and family. He was a very ordinary man living what most people would call a very ordinary life.

But he had one claim to fame. For five consecutive years he had won the blue ribbon in the Village Garden Show with his prize rose. It had gone on so long that people had come to expect it. John Deckard's prize rose would win, and that was that.

Behind his house was his rose garden. When he returned home each evening, he would don his coveralls and spend his time out there with his roses. Some said he had more than just "a way with flowers." Some said he mothered them, that he talked to them and that they understood what he said.

This year, deep in his own heart, John Deckard knew that he would again win the blue ribbon, for this year his rose was truly a rose among roses. Never had he seen such perfection in a flower. This was his masterpiece and as he watched it daily, his contentment and pride grew.

The show was on Saturday and he planned to transplant his rose to a pot early in the morning. But while he was at breakfast, the tragedy happened. His little son Rob burst into the kitchen, and chatting excitedly he rushed to the table and cried, "Look Daddy, look what I have for you!" And in his grimy little hand, half its petals gone, its head drooping, was John Deckard's prize rose.

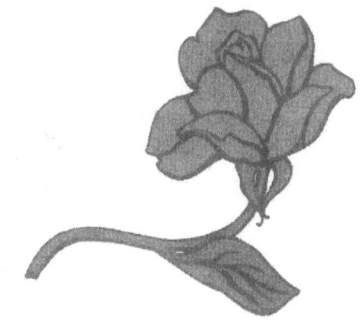

That afternoon, visitors to the Garden Show were astonished when they came to John Deckard's entry. For in a flower pot he had thrust a stick, and attached to it, at the very top, was a picture of his little son, Rob. When the judges heard what had happened, they gave John Deckard an honorary blue ribbon. Some said that the rose that was not a rose was the finest he had ever grown. God's love is like that and we can all be thankful.

A CHRISTION NEWS PAPER CUTTING

KEYS IN A FISH

I recently heard the story of a mother in an African nation who came to Christ, and grew strong in her commitment and devotion to the Lord. As so often happens, however, this alienated her from her husband, and over the years he grew to despise and hate her new devotion to Christ.

His anger and bitterness reached their climax when he decided to kill his wife, their two children and himself, unable to live in such self-inflicted misery. But he needed a motive. He decided that he would accuse her of stealing his precious keys - the keys were to the bank, the house, and the car. Early one afternoon he left his bank and headed for the tavern. His route took him across a footbridge extended over the headwaters of the Nile River. He paused above the river and dropped the keys. He spent all afternoon drinking and carousing.

Later that afternoon, his wife went to the fish market to buy the evening meal. She purchased a large Nile perch. As she was gutting the fish, to her astonishment in its belly were her husband's keys. How had they gotten there? What were the circumstances? She did not know; but she cleaned them up and hung them on the hook.

Sufficiently drunk, the young banker came home that night and pounded open the front door shouting, "Woman, where are my keys?" Already in bed, she got up, picked them off the hook in the bedroom, and handed them to her husband. When he saw the keys, by his own testimony he immediately became sober and was instantly converted. He fell on his knees, sobbing, asked for forgiveness, and confessed Jesus Christ as his Lord and Saviour.

IF JESUS CAME BACK

Would you have to change your clothes
Before you let Him in?
Or hide some magazines,
And put the Bible where they'd been?

Would you hide your worldly music
And put some hymn books out?
Could you let Jesus walk right in,
Or would you rush about?

And I wonder if the Saviour
Spent a day or two with you,
Would you go right on doing,
The things you always do?

Would you go right on saying
The things you always say?
Or would life for you continue
As it does from day to day?

Would you take Jesus with you
Everywhere you go?
Or would you maybe change your plans
For just a day or so?

Would you be glad to have Him
Meet your closest friends?
Or would you hope they stay away
Until His visit ends?

Would you be glad to have Him stay
Forever on and on?
Or would you sigh with great relief
When He at last was gone?

It might be interesting to know,
The things that you would do,
If Jesus came in person,
To spend some time with you.

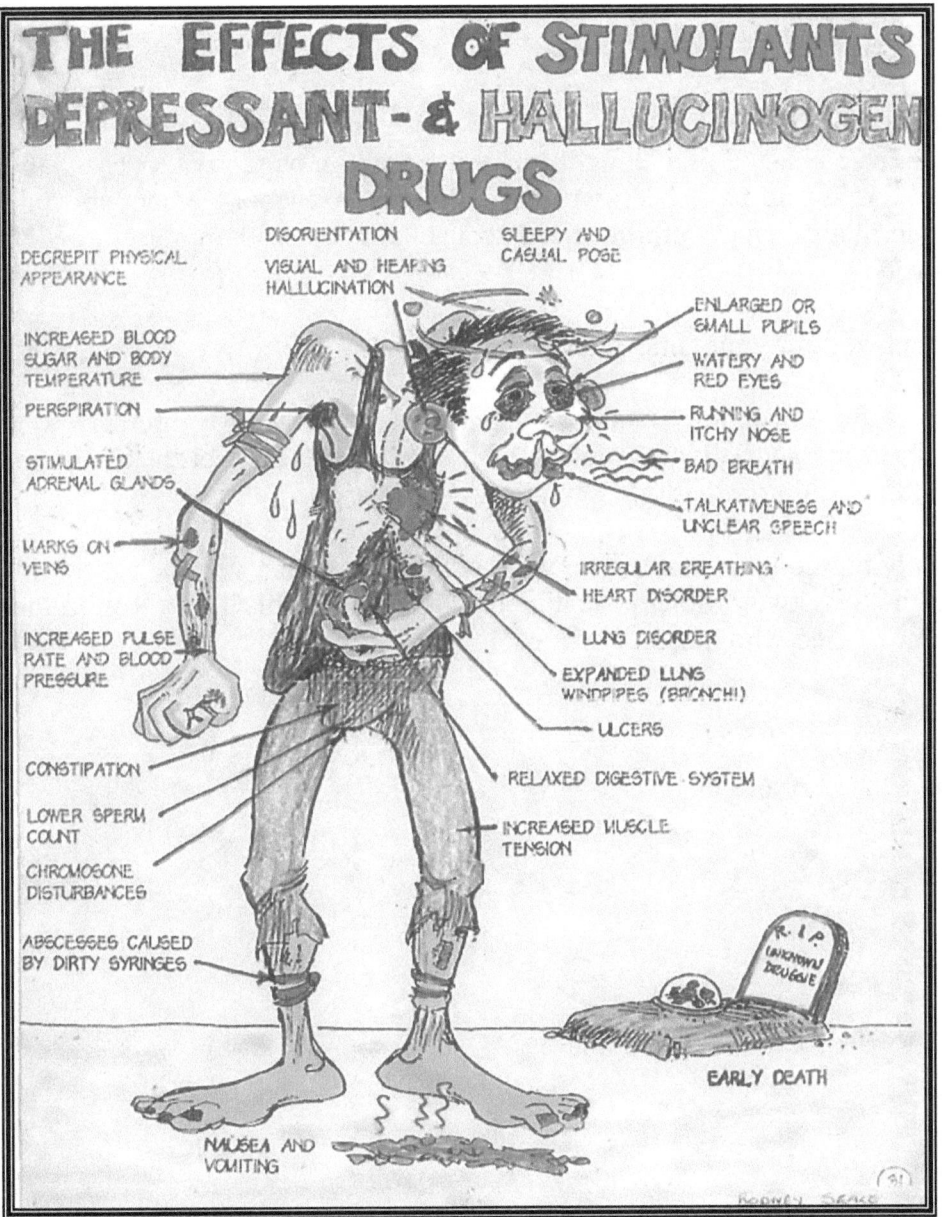

Thank you

To my family, those near, those far, those who have passed away, all who have assisted in making this life story put on paper, without you all, no book would have been written, no words of encouragement spoken, no spirit awakened to forge ahead against all odds, faith in myself, belief in you all.

Thank you for your contributions.

My wife, Martie for standing by, that helping had. My mother gave birth to me and I lived to tell all about it, Martie gave birth to all five children, Lillian, Charlotte, Quintin, Angelique and Patrick.

Lastly but no least those who were with me from the very beginning of my life, my two brothers, Austin and Mike, my family I love you in the name of God who made us all.

Amen.

Praise the Lord.

BIBLIOGRAPHY

1. The Bible
2. Atkins diet
3. Free State Tourism pamphlet
4. A devotional Diary—2 listeners-
5. Muscle evolution magazine
6. Cancer Association of SA
7. Dictionaries
8. Doctors books
9. Universal Newspaper
10. Hallmark connection: Greeting Workshop
11. CreataCard Gold 2
12. American Greeting CreataCard 7

www.ingramcontent.com/pod-product-compliance
Lightning Source LLC
Chambersburg PA
CBHW061257280526
45784CB00002B/794